# Fun on Foot in America's Cities

## Warwick Ford

*with* Nola Ford

Wyltan Books
Cambridge, Massachusetts, U.S.A.

This book is designed to help you make decisions regarding your fitness program. It is not intended as a substitute for professional fitness and medical advice. As with all fitness programs, you should seek your doctor's approval before you begin.

There are safety risks inherent in running, jogging, or walking in cities, and conditions can change. The publisher and authors are not responsible for harm to persons or property that results from use of the contents of this book.

Wyltan and Fun on Foot are trademarks of Wyltan, Inc.

ISBN 978-0-9765244-0-3   paperback
ISBN 0-9765244-0-6   paperback
Library of Congress Control Number: 2005907045

Printed in the United States of America by BookMasters, Inc.

Available in bookstores and online at http://www.funonfoot.com

Wyltan Books
Cambridge, Massachusetts, U.S.A.

This is a 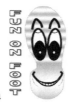 Book

# Table of Contents

# Preface

After spending many years on the road, trying to motivate myself to get out and jog around strange cities, I think I found the answer: Arm yourself with the information necessary to instantly locate outstandingly pleasant and enjoyable routes. Jogging around cities can be enormously rewarding, not just from the fitness viewpoint, but also from the perspective of getting to know a place and enjoying it.

I discussed the idea of a book on urban on-foot exercise routes with many people who travel, ranging from serious marathon runners through to people who just want to get out and walk a good distance. I concluded that the same collection of information would be useful to all of these people. Hence, this book is targeted equally at runners, joggers, and serious walkers.

I am delighted that my wife Nola also became hooked on this project. Today she agrees that her participation in researching this book is far and away the most valuable contribution to her fitness and her travel enjoyment in recent years.

Because the state of urban on-foot trails is changing so rapidly, we have launched a website along with this book, to distribute one-page printouts of routes and up-to-date information about the places covered. Please visit http://www.funonfoot.com for the latest updates, and to provide your feedback to the community.

An enormous number of people contributed in greater or lesser ways to this book. We talked to many people along the routes, while traveling to or from the cities, and in local bars and coffee shops. Staff of business establishments in the target cities also helped greatly.

The following people stand out for their special help in researching this project or reviewing the manuscript: Ric Bremer, Steven Cox, Jackie Cressy, Peter Cressy, Alex Deacon, Richard Fallon, Terry Ford, Charlie Geisz, Harry Greco, Carmel Haugh, Rob Kooney, Greg Mulligan,

Frank O'Neill, Donna Skultety, Dave Solo, and Allen Volchuk. Thank you all for your contributions and for sharing with us your knowledge of and familiarity with at least one of the cities.

I must especially recognize our daughter, Louisa, herself a dedicated runner, for her contributions in researching several routes, reviewing the manuscript, and helping with the photography.

Nola and I hope you will enjoy reading and using this book, and that it contributes in some little way to your future quality of life.

Warwick Ford
Cambridge, Massachusetts, U.S.A.

# Introduction

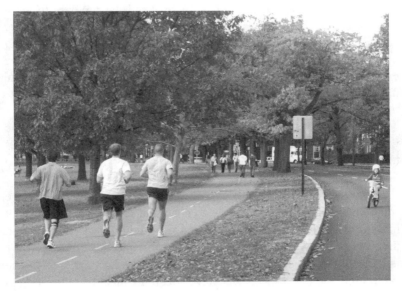

T his book is for people who like the idea of getting outdoors for some on-foot exercise, and either live in U.S. cities or travel to these cities for business or pleasure.

Most people would agree that on-foot exercise—running, jogging, or walking—is a really good thing. Any exercise unquestionably helps one control weight, increase life expectancy, feel more energetic, and look better. On-foot exercise has some particular attractions: It is inexpensive; it can be done almost anywhere and on your own schedule; it can be done alone or with company; and there are many ways to make it motivating and fun.

However, even those of us who really buy the idea of on-foot exercise will, all too often, admit we do not actually get out enough or keep going far enough. It is easy not to exercise.

I am convinced the main reason is that on-foot exercise is too often boring, devoid of attractions, and even downright uncomfortable. Many people really don't like emulating a hamster in an uninspiring, antisocial gym or hotel exercise room. Getting outdoors is much more pleasant and interesting. However, one is often unsure of where to go and what will be encountered on the way. In essence, on-foot exercise is, too often, just *not enough fun*. This makes it far too easy to resist carving out the necessary time from other activities that seem more comfortable and enjoyable, such as sitting around chatting, watching TV, and driving around in automobiles. Even work is all too often the excuse for not exercising. Hence, my most basic conclusion: One must always strive to make on-foot exercise fun. This is a key theme throughout this book.

A keen on-foot exerciser who has lived in a place a long time will know enjoyable on-foot routes there, having had the opportunity to explore the area, and to build familiarity and confidence in some favorite routes.

However, when new to an area or traveling, especially in a city, the situation is different. Most people do not find it easy to head out on foot in unfamiliar cities because of a shortage of the right information and the absence of a warm fuzzy feeling. The consequence: Forget it! Stay indoors, use the car, and worry about getting exercise another day. The same applies to many locals who have not quite found the motivation to seek out favorite outdoor on-foot routes in their hometowns.

In the case of America's cities, there is even a broad preconception that these are not generally good places to be outdoors on foot. On-foot exercise in cities is often considered to be an unpleasant and possibly even a dangerous activity.

As a seasoned traveler, I have experienced those feelings many times. I was a corporate road warrior for way too many years and I have always been a keen leisure traveler. However, I was lucky enough to have a few exceptional on-foot experiences on interesting routes in strange cities. This gave me cause to further explore how to make urban outdoor exercise motivating.

The first experience that stands out occurred several years ago, when I had a weekend business layover in downtown San Francisco. I was craving something healthy, energizing, and different to do. I became intrigued with the idea of jogging from Fisherman's Wharf to Sausalito across the Golden Gate Bridge. No guide books recommended this and my hotel concierge did not think it was feasible. However, I decided to give it a go. The result: The Bay was gorgeous; the bridge was far more awesome than it had ever been in a car; and there was an enormous amount to see. Finding the way into Sausalito was a little challenging. However, I ended up enjoying a beer, sandwich, and some memorable laughs with the locals in Sausalito, before catching the ferry back across the glorious bay. My feelings at the time were that this was the most enjoyable, exciting, and satisfying on-foot experience I had ever had.

As a result of that revelation, and many subsequent comparable experiences in other cities, I developed a new attitude. On-foot exercise in U.S. cities is not just OK but can be enormously enjoyable and rewarding from a range of perspectives. It can most definitely be *fun*. All one needs is some information up front, and this book aims to put that information in *your* hands.

I have a partner in crime who now needs to be introduced—my long-time wife and running mate, Nola. I rarely had the pleasure of her company during my business trips, but we have been a team in recent years for all the on-foot city explorations that provide the foundation for this book.

In this book I do not generally distinguish between running, jogging, and walking as forms of exercise. While faster exercise burns calories more quickly, all forms are good. Despite much time on foot, I am still abysmally slow, compared with any norm you might dream up. Nevertheless, jogging (many people would not grace my actions with the term *running*) is a key activity in preserving my fitness and keeping my weight down. On any given outing, Nola and I usually start out jogging. If either of our bodies starts to protest loudly enough along the way, we then fall back to walking. On other occasions, such as very hot days, we just decide at the outset to have a nice walk.

However, we always finish the route. We believe that is most important.

One thing that still surprises me is the number of people who are reluctant to try the routes described in this book saying, "I can't walk four miles, and certainly not ten!" When pressed to try, they almost always must retract those preconceptions. If you just give it a try, almost anyone without severe disabilities can walk four miles without pain in under an hour-and-a-half and ten miles in three hours or so.

If you are prepared to do some walking but will not run or jog at all, this book is still for you. You might be surprised at how rapidly your distances and times improve.

When I say walking, I mean walking at a good pace—not strolling. One of the main impediments we on-foot exercisers face is that person who strolls along at a snail's pace, blocking the sidewalk or pedestrian trail and making no attempt to get his or her blood pumping.

While slow pedestrians are a pain, there is one other entity that really is our Public Enemy Number 1: the *automobile*. The more we can tame our urge to get into that metal box, the more walking, jogging, or running we shall inevitably do. Therefore, when traveling, I do not like renting a car to drive somewhere to run an out-and-back loop from the car park. Since we can often survive and save our precious funds by not renting a car when traveling, I shall try to exclude automobile dependence throughout our travels in this book.

Enough of the preamble… Let us cut to the chase and spell out just where this book is going to take you. After my many years of skirting the fitness edge, I have become convinced that on-foot exercise becomes *enormously* more enjoyable if one ensures that the route chosen has four attributes: (1) comfort; (2) attractions; (3) convenience; and (4) a destination. Add to this a couple of other desirable but optional factors—such as good companionship and a nice day—and you are well on the way to more time out on foot.

Let me expand further on those four attributes of a route.

*Comfort*, which is the most essential attribute, has several elements, all of which are fairly obvious but worth noting. First, there should be minimal safety concerns. There should be a reasonable expectation that there will not be a nasty surprise around the next corner.[1] The number of other people around should be in your comfort zone (not too many and not too few). Underfoot conditions should also be reasonable, if not excellent. There should be a minimum of encounters with vehicular traffic.

---

1      See the table of violent crime statistics at the end of this chapter.

Comfort also depends on weather. Most people can run or jog comfortably at temperatures between 40 and 80 degrees Fahrenheit, and if you are very fit you can likely add some leeway to that. If you really feel it is too hot, still go out, but maybe earlier in the day or run less and walk more. Running or jogging in wet, icy, or snowy conditions is not a good idea because of the risk of injury.[2]

By *attractions* I mean that the route should be environmentally pleasant and interesting. It helps enormously if a route has points of historic or cultural interest, scenic beauty, or people activities on the day. In major cities, there tend to be more interesting things to see and more people activities. Therefore, on-foot routes in major cities can often be winners in this regard. To be interesting, variety is also fundamental. Any route can become boring with time, so it is good to have some elements to vary each time. Also, we like to avoid out-and-back routes. Repeating everything you saw in the first half of a route on the way back is somehow less satisfying than having something new to see all the way. Therefore, we try to create circular routes; if necessary, we fill in part of the loop by another form of transportation.

*Convenience* means ease of getting to the start of a route from a city's center or the areas where visitors tend to stay. Similarly, getting back from the end of a route should be easy. Given our belief that the number one enemy of on-foot fitness is the automobile, we try to avoid any need for use of an automobile in getting to, from, or along our routes. If other forms of transportation are required to close a loop, we look mainly to public transit, so as to minimize costs, hassle, and dependence on the automobile.

*Destination* is an important factor to many people but not everyone. Serious runners frequently gain their on-foot satisfaction from successfully meeting their own time and distance goals, and are then content to get straight back to their home or hotel for a shower. However, a lot of people struggle to get out on-foot and to complete a route of sufficient distance. Having a clear destination in mind helps make a route motivating and also reduces the temptation to quit early. If you are mentally on a mission to go somewhere enjoyable, then odds are you will make it there. Therefore, we consider it valuable to have

---

2        Throughout this book we quote average temperature and precipitation statistics for U.S. cities. These are from the Weatherbase website of Canty and Associates, LLC: www.weatherbase.com.

routes end up in places where there is something interesting to see or do afterwards, should one so choose.

Another aspect of a destination that helps many people is having a good food-beverage opportunity waiting at the end. Nola and I have found this works for us. When we first started pushing ourselves to run more, it became apparent that Nola was way more likely to start and complete an eight-mile weekend jog if there was a tasty brunch at the end. I was way more likely to do the same if there was a glass of cold beer at the end. Is it a bad thing to encourage people to run, jog, or walk to a place where they end up eating and drinking? Won't the damage done by the food and drinks cancel out the good done by the exercise? I think the answer to both questions is, "Not necessarily." You will probably eat anyway. Also, on-foot exercise is accompanied by heavy calorie burning (see the table *Estimated Calories Burned in a 5- or 10-mile Route*)[3]. Your calorie-count will end up in much better shape than if you were not exercising at all, giving more leeway for food consumption. Of course, moderation in quantity and judicious selection of nutritious foods should always be followed.

Since we believe there is a correlation between the set of people who really relish a good meal or drink and the set of people who most need more exercise, we do not feel anyone should shy away from the food-and-drink motivation angle. A little extra indulgence in the food and drink department is a perfectly reasonable inducement to exercise, especially if you *only* allow yourself the indulgence if you do the exercise first.

Consequently, one theme you will find in this book is the idea of ending each route near a good eating and drinking establishment, where you can wind down if you so choose. We tend to look for pub-restaurants—places that will happily accept people in running gear and a little sweaty. We look out, in particular, for top-notch Irish pubs that have interesting character, along with good food, drink, and company. That is not essential, though. There are many other quality

---

3        Figures computed from data in: Maria Adams, MS, MPH, RD, "The Benefits and Risks of Walking Versus Running," HealthGate http://www. somersetmedicalcenter.com/110324.cfm. Note, however, that calorie burn rate depends on many factors including, but not limited to, amount of skeletal muscle, running efficiency, speed, surface type, incline, resting metabolism, level of fitness, and outside temperature. (Thanks to Ayesha Rollinson for explaining this.) Therefore, consider the figures in the table as indicative only.

eating and drinking establishments in U.S. cities that satisfy the basic requirement.

If you have no need for food and drink exercise motivators, please ignore our references to restaurants and pubs.

| Body Weight: | 110 lb. (50 Kg.) | 150 lb. (68 Kg.) | 190 lb. (86 Kg.) |
|---|---|---|---|
| Walking 5 miles | 380 | 500 | 650 |
| Jogging 5 miles | 392 | 530 | 674 |
| Running 5 miles | 432 | 567 | 708 |
| Walking 10 miles | 760 | 1000 | 1300 |
| Jogging 10 miles | 783 | 1060 | 1348 |
| Running 10 miles | 864 | 1134 | 1416 |

**Estimated Calories Burned in a 5- or 10-mile Route**
Assumed speeds: Walking 3.0 mph, Jogging 5.2 mph, Running 7.5 mph

\* \* \* \*

Having pinned down all these important positive attributes of good on-foot routes, we decided to select several U.S. cities and try to find two or more routes in each that satisfy all of the criteria outlined above. In describing these routes, we also try to provide helpful information for those readers who want to devise their own routes in those cities, without necessarily following exactly what we lay out.

We selected 14 of the country's largest cities, taking into account the likelihood of satisfying our criteria. The list is as follows: Atlanta, Boston, Chicago, Dallas, Denver, Indianapolis, Los Angeles, Minneapolis, New York, Philadelphia, San Diego, San Francisco, Seattle, and Washington. We made a point of visiting each city and developing our ideas on foot. We tried and rejected many routes in many cities that did not meet all criteria. A few routes that we felt were just too good to miss we have flagged as *Fun on Foot Classic Routes*.

We generally restrict our route recommendations to the four-to-ten mile range, distances that are not too long for a half-day walk and long enough for a nice run for all but the serious distance runner.

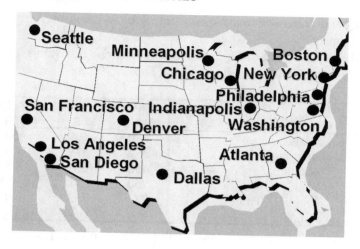

**Fun-on-Foot Cities**

Some readers will likely enjoy following the exact routes we suggest. However, that is certainly not essential and we expect many of you will take up some of the ideas we present and design your own enjoyable outings around them.

Since you may not want to carry this book around while out on foot, we have produced a one-page summary of each route, including map and directions. These summaries are available for printing from our website: http:// www.funonfoot.com.

If we missed your favorite city or route, I apologize for that. Please email us your ideas about other cities and routes—we shall take your ideas into account in a future book or revision of this one.

One question we often get is what about bikes? Why not cycle these routes? While cycling is a fine fitness activity, we just do not find it very practical when traveling. You are faced with such problems as obtaining a bike, leaving it somewhere safe when you want to go into a restaurant or shop, storing it in the evening, and getting it onto public transit (if that is even possible). Furthermore, we find that many attractive places that are ideal for running or walking do not permit cycling or are just not suitable for cycling. Therefore, while some of our routes use bicycle paths, we do not limit our routes to paths suitable for cycling and, as a consequence, can frequently offer on-footers a superior experience.

Inline skating is closer to on-foot exercise. Some but not all of our routes are suitable for inline skating. In each route description, we try to assess the extent to which inline skating will work.

On that note, let us conclude the lead-in and embark on our tour, focusing on urban on-foot routes with the comfort/attractions/convenience/destination formula as our guiding light. We shall start in the nation's northeast corner and work generally toward the southwest.

Our main message: Get out on foot, get fit, see interesting places, and—most importantly—have fun!

| City | Violent Criminal Offenses per 1,000 Inhabitants in 2003 |
|---|---|
| San Diego, CA | 5.8 |
| Denver, CO | 6.2 |
| Seattle, WA | 6.8 |
| New York, NY | 7.3 |
| San Francisco, CA | 7.4 |
| Indianapolis, IN | 8.8 |
| Minneapolis, MN | 11.9 |
| Boston, MA | 12.2 |
| Los Angeles, CA | 12.7 |
| Chicago, IL | 13.0 |
| Dallas, TX | 13.7 |
| Philadelphia, PA | 13.8 |
| Washington, DC | 15.7 |
| Atlanta, GA | 19.7 |

**Violent Crime Indexes for Cities Covered**
Source: FBI *Crime in the United States*, 2003

NOTE: Chicago figure may be lower than actual, since forcible rape was not reported.

| | |
|---|---|
| • • • • • • • | Recommended on-foot route |
| ▪ ▪ ▪ ▪ ▪ ▪ ▪ | Major highway |
| 🚌 | Public transit stop (Bus, rail, or subway) |
| 🚻 | Public restroom |
| 🚻 | Public restroom (Seasonal) |
| 🥤 | Drinking water |
| 🥤 | Drinking water (Seasonal) |

Omitted on water-plentiful routes

| | |
|---|---|
| 🍷 | Casual eating/drinking establishment with good food, suitable for terminating an athletic route |
| 1 | Point of interest |

## Key to Map Symbols

# 2

# Beantown

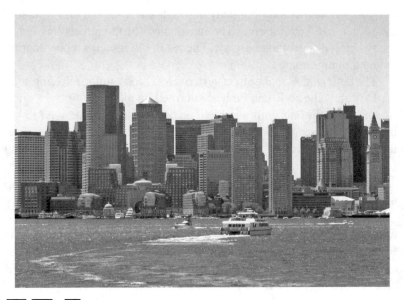

W e begin our tour in Boston, Massachusetts—point of the nation's conception.  This is where plotting for the American Revolution was centered.  Boston is or was the home of Paul Revere, Samuel Adams (both the revolutionary and the beer company), the Red Sox, the New England Patriots, and the nation's best collection of Irish Pubs.

Boston also happens to have been my and Nola's home base for several years, so we can speak with real authority about this place.

Boston is a city of the young (the region is host to way more than its fair share of the nation's top colleges) and the young at heart.  This makes it a dream city for jogging, running, or walking.  There is a massive foot-mobile population, so if you feel like a jog anywhere here you will never feel out of place and rarely be on your own. Do not feel pressured to limit your running to parks or reserves. Running through the streets of downtown Boston or adjacent Cambridge is a perfectly normal activity.

In fact, travel by foot is an important mode of transport in Boston. One reason is the city's compactness, making it easy to negotiate on foot. The more compelling reason, however, is that the traffic system is so dysfunctional many people think twice about driving anywhere in central Boston or Cambridge. The street layout was never planned but just grew higgledy-piggledy through the roughly 400 years of the settlements' evolution. The narrowness of the streets has led to many being designated one-way. The result often seems a bewildering navigation nightmare.

The deficiencies in the street system have bred a unique driving style for Boston. The style can be best summed up as *anything goes*, short of actually colliding with a vehicle or pedestrian. If you *need* to get into a traffic stream from a blind-intersection side street you just push into that traffic stream. If you *need* to turn left in face of approaching traffic to keep your stream moving, you turn left. Furthermore, drivers tend not to let little things like stop signs and red lights hold them up unnecessarily.

However, Boston drivers are generally very alert, defensive, and more-or-less unflappable. Many out-of-towners (especially people from New York where horn-tooting is mandatory every 10 seconds) are amazed at the scarcity of horn tooting in Boston, given the wild and creative driving acts that continually happen.

The driving attitude flows through to pedestrians as well. If you *need* to cross a busy street, you just have to assert yourself and cross it. Drivers are generally kind to pedestrians and will usually stop for them without getting particularly upset. (Don't take me too literally on this one, though. You need to develop just the right pedestrian judgment for Boston.)

This type of driving and pedestrian behavior is virtually essential if the people of Boston are to get anywhere at all.

Travel by foot is quite common. For example, Nola and I think nothing of walking the roughly three miles from our Cambridge home to Fenway Park to see a Red Sox game, or to the downtown Boston shops, pubs, and restaurants.

The other alternative to driving is the T—Boston's public transit system that comprises a mixture of subways, light rail, and buses. The T, launched in 1897, was the first U.S. subway system and is the fourth oldest in the world

Unfortunately, the T is something of an embarrassment to us Bostonians. It looks dreadful, in comparison to the transit systems in most other cities. In fact, an observer from a faraway galaxy could be excused for concluding that the main purpose of the system is to transport trash around the city, while passengers squeeze on if there is room. Nevertheless, the T is convenient, efficient, and generally devoid of the surprises we have encountered in certain other cities' transit systems.

\* \* \* \*

Boston's weather is quite good for running. The average daily maximum is in our preferred 40-to-80 degrees range all months except January (36°), February (38°), and July (82°). There can be snow or ice underfoot in December through March, so running might be out then. It rarely gets too hot to run; the worst you might have to do is start out early on a hot summer day. There is precipitation on average 126 days of the year so there is some risk this might ruin your day out on foot.

As to street safety, Boston has a violent crime index of 12.2 (violent crimes per 1,000 inhabitants in 2003). This is a little over the average for all cities covered in this book. We shall try to exclude areas with bad reputations from our routes, but we must caution you that this matter is ultimately your own responsibility. Please always use good street sense.

\* \* \* \*

Now, let us try to pin down the best on-foot exercise routes convenient to central Boston. There is one no-brainer. The lower Charles River between Boston and Cambridge is one of the best and most popular running, jogging, and walking areas in the country. We have built our prime route there, also linking up with Boston's most historical precincts. After that, we have selected some other routes that take in the Charles River further upstream, the Emerald Necklace to Jamaica Plain, the oceanfront, and the Neponset River, south of downtown. We believe we have nailed the best routes conveniently accessible from downtown.

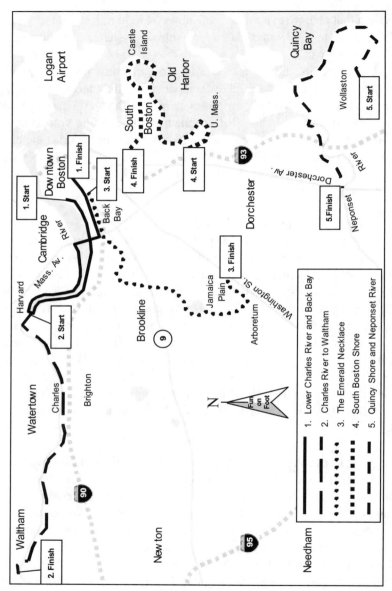

**Boston Routes**

| Route | Distance |
|---|---|
| 1. Lower Charles River and Back Bay | 8.7 miles |
| 2. Charles River to Waltham | 7.0 miles |
| 3. The Emerald Necklace | 6.7 miles |
| 4. South Boston Shore | 7.9 miles |
| 5. Quincy Shore and Neponset River | 6.5 miles |

# Lower Charles River and Back Bay

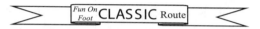

| Distance | 8.7 miles (can cut to 4.4 miles) |
|---|---|
| Comfort | Excellent running conditions. Plenty of on-foot exercisers around. Crowds are unlikely to be a concern unless you hit a special event. OK for inline skating. |
| Attractions | Pass by or near several city sights, including the Hatch Shell, MIT, Harvard University, Trinity Church, and the old Granary Burial Ground. Most of the route follows a very pleasant riverside pedestrian/bicycle trail and the rest is along wide, runner-friendly streets. |
| Convenience | Start at the T Red Line Charles/MGH station, a short walk or T ride from the financial district, Cambridgeside, and Kendall Square. End at Boston Common, close to historic sites, downtown shops, the financial district, theatre district, Copley Place, Hynes Convention Center, and the T Red Line Park station. Alternatively, the 4.4-mile shortened route ends at Harvard Square in Cambridge, near the T Red Line Harvard station. |
| Destination | Boston Common, the launch point for Boston's historic Freedom Trail, near downtown shops and some excellent restaurants and pubs for winding down. The 4.4-mile variation ends at lively Harvard Square, the center of the Harvard community, with shops, restaurants, and pubs. |

Our first route centers on the Charles River, combined with Back Bay. This is one of our hometown favorite routes. It scores high on all the attributes of comfort, attractions, convenience, and destination. While we describe one particular eight-mile route, you can easily adjust it to better fit your personal tastes if desired.

This route uses the Dr. Paul Dudley White Bicycle Path, a loop stretching from the Charles River Dam upstream nine miles to Watertown on both sides of the Charles River. It is (very appropriately) dedicated to the "Father of Modern Cardiology," one of Boston's famous sons (1886-1973).

The whole route is sealed. However, for much of its length you will find well-traveled dirt side paths or grassy verges that make it very runner-friendly. Restroom facilities are scarce; in fact the only one is at the Hatch Shell. There are a few water fountains (see the map) but they are disabled from late fall through early spring.

Our route starts at the Boston end of the Longfellow Bridge, named after Henry Wadsworth Longfellow, Maine-born, but generally considered one of Boston's favorite sons. This spot is not far from hotels in downtown Boston and eastern Cambridge. If you are not within walking distance, take the T Red Line to the Charles/MGH station.

Cross the footbridge to the river bank, then head upstream (in a southwesterly direction) on the Boston side of the river. The other side of the river is all part of Cambridge, with its diverse population heavy in students and academics.

The first notable place you pass is Community Boating. This is where Bostonians (Nola and I included) learn to sail. The swirling winds in the Charles Basin, coming off the nearby downtown high-rises, present ever variable, challenging, and fun sailing conditions. The objective is to venture forth in a 15-foot centerboard boat and avoid getting dunked in the dirty Charles.[1]

The riverside path takes you through Boston's best-known outdoor recreational area, the Esplanade. This nicely landscaped park is home to many community events.

A little south of Community Boating, you come to the Edward M. Hatch Memorial Shell, a major outdoor entertainment site, and the center of such outstanding events as the July 4 and December 31 fireworks

---

1        A visitor can buy a part-year membership of Community Boating or just walk in with the hope of hitching a free joyride with a local sailor.

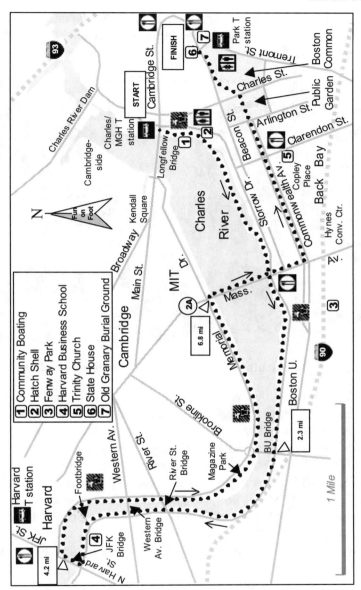

displays, to the accompaniment of the Boston Pops. This is also where many organized runs and walks start or end. On the opposite bank of the Charles is Massachusetts Institute of Technology (MIT), world-leading engineering and science school.

Cross the footbridge and pass the sculpture of the head of Arthur Fiedler, renowned and beloved conductor of the Boston Pops for fifty years.

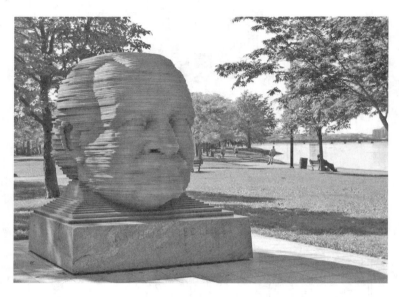

**Arthur Fiedler Sculpture with the Charles River Trail at Right**

Continuing up the river, at 1.2 miles from the Longfellow Bridge you encounter the next bridge, whose name is a source of never-ending confusion. It is officially named the Harvard Bridge, having been dedicated to Reverend John Harvard. Unfortunately, it is nowhere near Harvard University. In fact, its Cambridge endpoint is right in the middle of MIT, so some people call it the MIT Bridge. Because the road it carries is Mass. Av. (you would never, ever speak out the full "Massachusetts Avenue" words in Boston), we shall call it the Mass. Av. Bridge. This is the name every local will instantly understand.

While you have various route choices at this point, we suggest continuing upstream on the Boston side.

The stretch up to the Boston University (BU) Bridge is pleasant. The pedestrian path takes you under the BU Bridge on a short boardwalk. Note there is not a convenient link from the river path to the bridge so no opportunity to cross the river here.

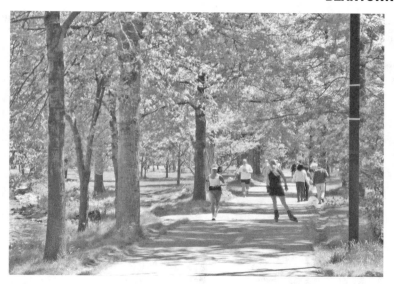

**Charles River Trail Near the Esplanade**

You are now in the vicinity of Boston University, the fourth largest independent university in the United States. On the opposite bank are the western parts of MIT.

The conditions after the BU Bridge are less than perfect, comprising mainly a paved bicycle path adjacent to busy Storrow Drive. However, the scenery along the river is still pleasant. Roughly a mile from the BU Bridge is the River Street Bridge, the first place you need to stop for cars. Cross River Street at the pedestrian crossing. At this point, you could cross the river and head back downstream, but we recommend going further upstream.

The Western Avenue Bridge is a quarter mile from the River Street Bridge. Cross Western Avenue. You now enter Harvard territory and conditions improve greatly in all respects. Harvard University, established in 1636, claims to be the first college established in North America. Continuing upstream, as you approach the Harvard footbridge (more correctly the John W. Weeks pedestrian bridge), you see on your left the Harvard Business School. This is where Lou Gerstner, Michael Bloomberg, and George W. Bush obtained their MBAs—whereas, across the river, Bill Gates dropped out of his undergraduate program as a junior. (If you ever become bored running, there lies a fertile topic for contemplation.)

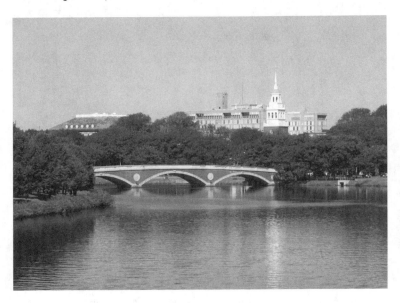

### The Charles River at Harvard

We suggest crossing the river at the next bridge, which links the Allston and Cambridge campuses of Harvard. This bridge is formally named the Larz Anderson Bridge, in recognition of a local political and diplomatic figure (1866-1937). However, locals will more likely recognize it as the JFK Bridge since, on the Cambridge side, it feeds JFK Street at JFK Memorial Park.

---

**VARIATION**

If you want to extend our route by two miles, continue upstream roughly a mile and cross the river at the Eliot Bridge. There is a water fountain there, and on-foot conditions are good throughout. Then continue back downstream to Harvard on the Cambridge side.

---

At the Cambridge end of the JFK Bridge, you are just a few short blocks from Harvard Square, the center of the Harvard campus and community.

---

**VARIATION**

If you only want a four-mile outing, you can stop here. There are many eating and drinking places, ranging from student joints to quality restaurants. For the on-footer we can recommend: John Harvard's Brewery (Dunster Street, one block east of JFK Street near Mount Auburn Street, with its own brews and great food); Legal Seafood at the Charles Hotel (Eliot Street, one block west of JFK, with great seafood and a casual bar/bistro atmosphere); and Grendel's Den (on the left side of JFK Street at Winthrop Street, a down-home pub for all ages with a wide selection of inexpensive food). You can then explore the Harvard campus and the nearby bookstores and museums. Return to downtown Boston via the T Red Line from Harvard Station at the north end of JFK Street.

---

From the Cambridge end of the JFK Bridge, head downstream on the Cambridge side of the Charles following Memorial Drive. It is 2.6 miles back to the Mass. Av. Bridge. The stretch from Harvard past the footbridge to the Western Avenue Bridge is particularly pleasant on Sundays from mid-spring to mid-fall, since Memorial Drive is closed to traffic. After that you pass the River Street Bridge. You then pass Magazine Park and come to a large rotary with an overpass for Memorial Drive traffic. Keep hard right and you pass the Cambridge end of the BU Bridge. Don't cross that bridge. Rather, continue downstream on the paved trail across the rail tracks. Note that the steps down towards the river here lead to a dead-end.

You will probably notice considerable wildlife on this part of the river. There is a substantial population of Canada Geese and ducks, and various other bird life depending on the time of year. However, one bird family that is somewhat unique is the flock of white geese that live year-round on the Cambridge side of the Charles, right around here. The flock numbers 60-plus birds and is generally loved by the local community.

One encounter with these birds sticks in my mind. I was running down the Charles at a time when the entire flock decided, for a reason known only to them, to cross busy Memorial Drive. One could well imagine a quite nasty mess, with more white feathers in the air than you would need to fill down comforters for a football squad. However, the process played out extraordinarily smoothly, thanks to the Boston driving attitude. The heavy traffic stopped and waited calmly while the 70-odd-bird flock waddled across the road, without a single feather flying or single honk from either birds or cars. Maybe more cities should adopt the Boston driving attitude…

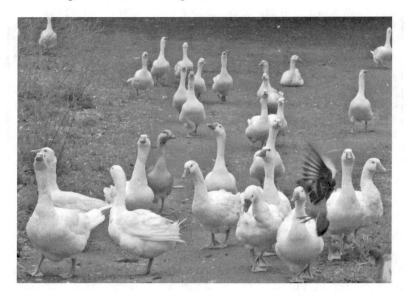

**The Cambridge White Geese Greet Visitors**

Continuing down the river, you come to a busy intersection with a traffic signal, at the Cambridge end of the Mass. Av. Bridge. This is very close to the center of MIT but, unless you have a specific objective, there is little point wandering through the MIT campus or trying to find good eating or drinking places thereabouts. We suggest you head back across the Charles at this point via the Mass. Av. Bridge and Route 2A to Back Bay.

Back Bay is a rare exception to Boston's confusing streets tradition, with its streets following an organized rectangular grid. This is because Back Bay did not even exist until the mid-1800s, when the city's leaders launched an ambitious 30-year program to landfill the marshlands on the south bank of the Charles River adjacent to downtown.

Our on-foot route continues to the historic part of Boston. However, if you wanted to stop earlier, you will find a range of good eating and drinking places throughout Back Bay. The first encountered that we would recommend is the Crossroads Pub, an Irish pub on Beacon Street

50 yards west of Mass. Av. Its pub food, drinks, and service are very good. This place also claims to be Back Bay's oldest pub, established immediately at the end of prohibition.

To continue, keep on Mass. Av. to the third light, then take a left along the center path of the Commonwealth Avenue Mall. This is a beautiful street—a 100-foot wide strip with generous pedestrian space, light vehicle traffic, and pleasant surrounds. The buildings were constructed in the latter half of the nineteenth century as Back Bay evolved through the filling-in of the marshlands. Originally these buildings were single-family residences. In the twentieth century, many were converted to condominiums or commercial use, but the overall external architecture and atmosphere have been preserved largely intact.

You will encounter several interesting statues and memorials along this eight-block route. For example, the Boston Women's Memorial recognizes three of Boston's famous daughters—Abigail Adams, Lucy Stone, and Phillis Wheatley—who, through their writings, made major contributions to social change.

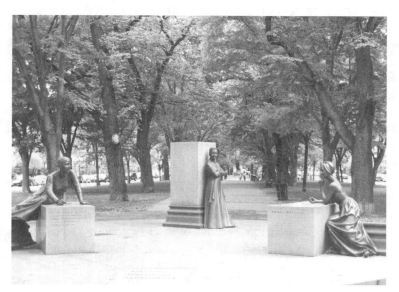

**Commonwealth Avenue Trail and the Boston Women's Memorial**

You cross several lightly trafficked streets. You might consider ending your route at Clarendon Street since, if you turn right here, you come to one of Back Bay's most famous buildings, Trinity Church, consecrated in 1876. The history of efforts to keep this entire beautiful establishment above the water level makes interesting reading. Also, across Clarendon Street from Trinity Church, there is a great seafood restaurant that is our top recommendation for Sunday Brunch in this part of Boston. Skipjack's excellent Sunday seafood brunch includes a jazz accompaniment. It is a teensy bit up-market, so bear that in mind when launching into here in your running gear. However, it has a bar area that comfortably accommodates all comers.

To continue to the end of our route, keep on Commonwealth Avenue to its termination at Arlington Street and the Boston Public Garden. Cross Arlington Street and enter the garden, passing Washington's statue. Cycling and inline skating are not permitted in the garden, but all forms of on-foot exercise are. Cross the footbridge over the swan boat rides (cute but not very helpful to your fitness). Continue straight through the garden to Charles Street and cross that street.

You then enter Boston Common, America's first public park, established in 1634. The Public Garden and Boston Common are lovely places for wandering and people watching but not a great running environment because of the crowds. Therefore, consider this a nice wind-down stretch.

Take the left path, northeastward through the Boston Common to Beacon Street. Continue to the Massachusetts State House, whose gold-leaf dome you cannot miss. This point, the nominal end point of our route, is also the start of Boston's Freedom Trail, the red sidewalk-marked trail that leads you through Boston's most famous historic sites.

Although Nola and I have run the Freedom Trail a couple of times, we do not recommend that because of the many slow people and the temptation to stop and look at things yourself. Consider it a sightseeing walk. To get started, follow Park Street to Tremont Street (Boston's original name was Tremontaine, reflecting the three hills that once dominated the landscape here). Turn left into Tremont Street and you come to the first major Freedom Trail site—the Old Granary Burial Ground, where Samuel Adams, John Hancock, and Paul Revere rest.

If you are ready for a food or drink break, there are many good establishments around here. We can recommend two top-class Irish pub/restaurants nearby. The first is Emmett's, a little further along Beacon Street from the State House, near Tremont Street. The food and décor are excellent and brunch is served on Saturday and Sunday.

For our other recommendation, head north on Tremont Street, which leads into Cambridge Street. Across from City Hall in Cambridge Street is the Kinsale Irish Pub & Restaurant, which has a genuine Celtic décor, good food and beer, and entertainment most evenings and for Sunday brunch.

Some other major Freedom Trail attractions are nearby. The Old State House is on State Street, off Cambridge Street near City Hall. Faneuil Hall (which, for the enlightenment of our French-speaking Canadian compatriots, is pronounced *fan-yul* hall) is just north of City Hall. Recognized as America's *Cradle of Liberty*, Faneuil Hall served as a central location for organizing protests against the British prior to the Revolution.

There are several other notable pub/restaurants nearby on the Freedom Trail. They include the Bell in Hand, which claims to be the oldest tavern in the country, with a history back to 1795, and the Union Oyster House, the oldest restaurant in Boston, established in 1826 in a building with a history back to 1742.

There are many more historic sites near here, and tacking some more sedate tourist activities onto the end of a good Charles River and Back Bay run, jog, or walk can mean an enormously satisfying day.

\* \* \* \*

You might wonder how Boston gained the moniker *Beantown*. It seems that, in colonial days, a favorite Boston food was beans baked in molasses for several hours.

# Charles River to Waltham

| | |
|---|---|
| **Distance** | 7.0 miles |
| **Comfort** | Paved dedicated pedestrian/bicycle trail all the way, with a dirt runner's side trail in places. Some parts follow road edges, but there is generally plenty of greenery and shade. Expect to pass the occasional other pedestrian or cyclist but don't expect crowds, except possibly along the first stretch in Cambridge. Not suitable for inline skating in parts. |
| **Attractions** | A pleasant escape from the hordes in central Boston. There is considerable wildlife along the river and nice scenery. Waltham is known for the Waltham Watch Company, a key innovator in the Industrial Revolution. |
| **Convenience** | Start at the JFK Bridge in Cambridge, near the T Red Line Harvard station and Harvard hotels. Finish in Waltham Center, where you can catch frequent buses (route 70/70A) back to the T Red Line Central station in Cambridge, or (less frequent) Commuter Rail to Boston's North Station. From Central or North Station you can take the T direct to all hotels. |
| **Destination** | The attractive riverside city center of Waltham. There is at least one excellent wind-down pub/restaurant here, and the Charles River Museum of Industry (open limited hours). |

If you liked the lower stretch of the Charles River, there is more enjoyment in store upstream from Harvard. There is a dedicated, paved trail extending upstream to Waltham, a historic city with a riverside city center. This route is different in character from our first route. It is much closer to the wilderness, giving better escape from the city environment for much of its length. It is also less used than the trail downstream from Harvard; so don't expect all the company you had there.

We have laid out this route as starting from the Larz Anderson Bridge (JFK Bridge) near Harvard. You can easily get here on the T Red Line to Harvard or, if you wish, travel on foot 4.2 miles from downtown Boston, following our first route.

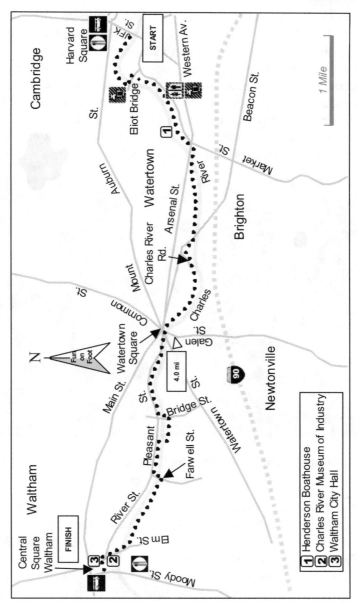

For the first four miles, from Harvard to Watertown Square, you can choose to follow either bank of the river. I shall recommend my preferred sides.

Start on the Cambridge side, following the river upstream to the next bridge, Eliot Bridge. This stretch is particularly pleasant on Sundays mid-spring to mid-fall, when Memorial Drive is closed to vehicles. Then cross Eliot Bridge on its left sidewalk, double back down to the river trail and use the pedestrian tunnel to cross under the road. Continue into and through a very pleasant part of the Charles River Reserve. Pass the canoe rentals, a playground with restrooms and water fountain, and the Northeastern University Henderson Boathouse. Continue to the Arsenal Street Bridge and cross the road here.

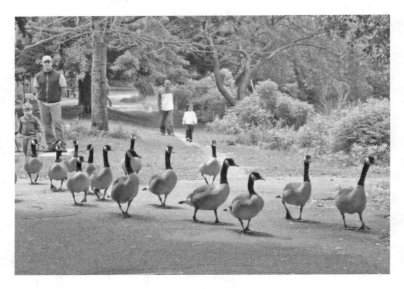

**Wildlife and People Sharing the Charles Trail Upstream from the Eliot Bridge**

For the segment from Arsenal Street Bridge to Watertown Square, the northern side is the better, with a dirt pedestrian trail plus a shared paved trail for much of the way. Cross the river on the Arsenal Street Bridge and pick up the trail upstream.

Cross Beacon Street at the next bridge, then head north along the paved sidewalk trail. Charles River Road splits off to the left towards the riverbank. Follow the trail along it. You are soon presented with some pleasant options, such as an unpaved pedestrian trail close to the river for much of the way.

Continue to Galen Street at Watertown Square. Cross Galen Street. There are restaurants and fast food joints around Watertown Square and you can catch the Route 70/70A bus back to Cambridge if you do not want to go further upstream. However, we encourage you to push on, as the trail conditions improve now.

Continuing upstream from Watertown Square, you can start on either side of the river. The south side trail will lead you to a footbridge to the north side anyway, so you might as well start on the north side. The conditions from here up to Waltham are excellent for on-foot exercise. The trails follow the river—not the roads. There is plenty of greenery, shade, and wildlife. However, civilization is never far away—you catch glimpses of residences and local businesses through the trees.

You have to switch banks of the river a few times and—be warned—the signage is poor. Follow the trail to where it emerges on Bridge Street. Then cross the river to the south bank and follow the streets around until you find a little trailhead that takes you back to the river. Midway along this next stretch, a footbridge takes you back to the north bank. Follow the trail to where it next emerges on Farwell Street. Cross the river back to the south side here, and pick up the trail again along that bank.

After going under the old railway bridge, the trail delivers you out on Elm Street. The riverbank path stops here. Follow Elm Street to the right. It leads you into Waltham Central Square, where you can stroll, admire the City Hall, and find food and drink places nearby.

Waltham was first settled in 1634 and was officially incorporated in 1738. It is known as Watch City, because the American Waltham Watch Company, one of the pioneers of the Industrial Revolution, operated here from 1854 to 1957. It was the first company to make watches on an assembly line.

Bus and Commuter Rail stops are in Waltham Central Square. However, the commercial center of Waltham is a short distance away. Go to the west side of the square then turn left, following Moody Street back across the river. The riverbank here is nicely landscaped, with a little walking path to the west. There is also a path to the east that takes you to the Charles River Museum of Industry, in the 1814-vintage Boston Manufacturing Company textile mill. This building is on the National Register of Historic Places as America's first factory. Be warned it only opens limited days though.

Possibly even more enticing are the shops and other establishments on Moody Street south of the river. If you feel like a really great place to wind-down for food and drinks, we can heartily recommend the Skellig Irish Pub. It has excellent food, including a brunch menu on Saturday and Sunday.

Backtrack to Waltham Central Square to catch public transit home. This route makes for a really great day's outing!

# The Emerald Necklace

| Distance | 6.7 miles |
|---|---|
| Comfort | Mostly excellent on-foot conditions under shady trees. There is some need to cross and follow trafficked streets. Expect a number of other on-foot exercisers around but crowds are unlikely to be a concern. Some parts are questionable for inline skating. At the end of the route, do not stray too far south or east since there lie some of Boston's more questionable areas. |
| Attractions | Experience some very attractively landscaped parks and trails close to central Boston. Escape completely from the bustle and the traffic in some parts. |
| Convenience | Start in Back Bay, handy to Red and Green Line T stations and hotels in the financial district, theatre district, Copley Place, or Hynes Convention Center vicinity. End at the T Orange Line Green Street station. The Orange line takes you direct to Back Bay, Hynes Convention Center, Copley Place, theatre district, financial district, and northern suburbs. |
| Destination | Doyle's Café, one of Boston's most famous Irish establishments with good food, drinks, and company. |

The Emerald Necklace extends from Back Bay to Jamaica Plain. Frederick Law Olmsted, designer of New York's Central Park, created the Emerald Necklace circa 1875. The overall plan involved a string of nine arguably contiguous "parks" stretching roughly eight miles in all. We have already covered the first three of these "parks"—the Boston Common, the Public Garden, and Commonwealth Avenue Mall—all of which predated Olmsted.

Olmsted's plan tacked on a string of further parks, following the course of the Muddy River, a stream feeding the Charles River. The Muddy River was long an embarrassment to Boston's inhabitants—a smelly, marshy annoyance. One of Olmsted's missions was to hide the Muddy River. He largely succeeded with that, although its unpleasantness still shows through when you get close enough at various spots today.

Heading progressively upstream, Olmsted's parks include the Back Bay Fens, the Riverway, Olmsted Park, Jamaica Pond, the Arnold Arboretum, and Franklin Park.

Running the course of these Muddy River parks is generally very pleasant; although you will need to cross a few busy roads *en route*. You probably do not want to go as far as Franklin Park, which does not have the best of reputations. Rather, we suggest ending the route at or just after the Arboretum.

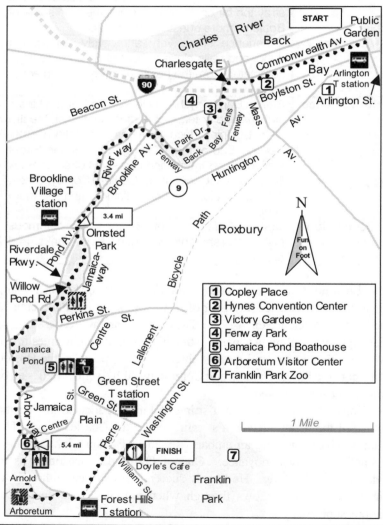

Start on Commonwealth Avenue in Back Bay, nominally at Arlington Street near the Public Garden. You can easily get here from the T Red Line Park station or Green Line Arlington station. Alternatively, if you are staying near Copley Place or the Hynes Convention Center, take the nearest northbound street up to Commonwealth Avenue.

Follow Commonwealth Avenue westbound, backtracking what we described in our first route. Cross Mass. Av., avoiding the underpass and keeping to the left, or southern, sidewalk. At Charlesgate E, turn left and take the sidewalk up the road ramp that emerges here. Go over Interstate 90 and cross Boylston Street at the light at the top of the ramp. You see Fenway Park, home of the Red Sox, away on your right. You also come to a sign announcing the start of the Back Bay Fens.

Enter the park and find yourself amidst a very impressive collection of community gardens. The centerpiece of this area is the Richard D. Parker Memorial Victory Garden. These gardens represent the last remaining of the region's victory gardens created during World War II. At that time, demands for food exports to the nation's armed forces in Europe and the Pacific caused rationing and shortages for those back home in the States. In response, President Roosevelt called for Americans to grow more vegetables. The City of Boston established 49 areas (including the Boston Common and the Public Gardens) as "victory gardens" for citizens to grow vegetables and herbs.

Today, these gardens are something special. Most are nurtured for their natural beauty more so than for bearing vegetables or flowers to cut and take away. Local individuals and families spend countless hours creating their own decorative piece of a remarkable landscape. There are various routes through the Back Bay Fens and their gardens, so take your pick.

The area is bounded on the left by Fenway and on the right by Park Drive. As you emerge from the Fens area you find yourself on one of these streets, which lead to a major intersection involving both Boylston Street and Brookline Avenue.

This "intersection" is a traffic nightmare for drivers, let alone us poor pedestrians. You need to cross the "intersection" in a generally northerly direction from where the Fens end. We recommend getting to the left, or outermost, side of Fenway before or at the first traffic signal. Cross Brookline Avenue and follow Fenway's left side into the bend where it changes name to Riverway. Cross the street at the marked pedestrian crossing. The main advice is to avoid getting into the center traffic island areas after Brookline Avenue since, despite the existence of pedestrian crossings; it is hard to get safely to where you want to go.

Sanity returns when you find the trailhead and sign welcoming you to the Riverway.

Along the Riverway, on-foot conditions are excellent. There are trails along both sides of the watercourse. We prefer the left (southeastern) side, which is unpaved and generally devoid of cyclists who prefer the other side that is paved. The left side is also further away from the sometimes-invasive T Green Line. You are treated to various interesting environmental enhancements, such as stone bridges and other structures, thanks to Mr. Olmsted's artistic ingenuity.

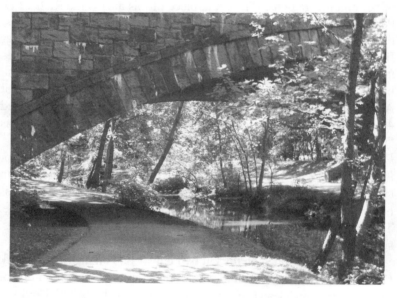

**The Riverway Trail and an Example of Olmsted's Stone Bridge Structures**

The first busy street you need to cross is Brookline Avenue. After crossing it, bear right following the tree-lined trail along its south side. Continue past Brookline Ice & Coal to where Brookline intersects Route 9. Cross the latter at the light. On the south side of Route 9, head back east a couple of hundred yards and find Pond Street and the sign welcoming you to Olmsted Park.

Olmsted Park has nicely varied terrain, with its share of wilderness areas and attractive landscaping. There are various ways through the park. You can bear right and follow a paved trail. This trail splits into separate pedestrian and bicycle tracks for much of the way. Alternatively, if you start off bearing left, you can pick up an unpaved trail through the middle of the park. This trail and a little network of dirt paths that link to it are particularly pleasant since they give you complete escape from traffic and most of the people. Yet another alternative is to keep bearing hard left, where there is a paved path following Jamaicaway down the east edge of the park.

Whichever path you choose, proceed south to Willow Pond Road, cross it and continue south to Perkins Street. Cross Perkins Street and you come to Jamaica Pond—a large, circular and very pleasant pond, with a 1.5-mile pedestrian and bicycle path around it. You can go around the pond either way. The more pleasant option is to bear to the right, and go around the pond counterclockwise. However, if you need to use facilities, go the clockwise direction; this takes you past the Jamaica Pond Boat House where there are restrooms and a water fountain.

Continue to the south end of the lake where you see a road curving off towards the southwest, as part of a larger system of roads to the south. This is Arborway, the road system connecting Jamaica Pond and the Arnold Arboretum. Take the right hand sidewalk along Arborway to a large rotary, admiring the charming houses along the way. Follow the edge of the rotary around to the right, crossing Centre Street (yes, it really is spelt that way). Despite the marked pedestrian crossing adjacent to the rotary, you might find it difficult crossing here; if so, go 100 yards up Centre Street and cross at the light.

Now follow the road around to the southeast away from the rotary (the road is still called Arborway here, or Route 203). After a short distance, you come to the main entrance to the Arboretum.

Vehicles are generally excluded from the Arboretum, so it is a pedestrian's delight. There are wide roads and paths to follow, with plenty of room for runners, joggers, walkers, and plant gazers alike. Admission is free.

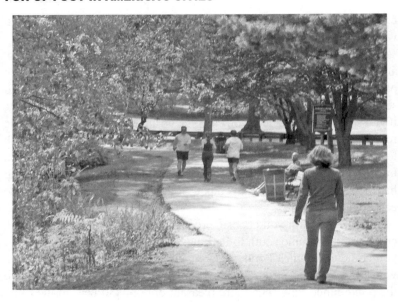

## The Trail Around Jamaica Pond

Inside this entrance to the right is the Hunnewell Building, housing a Visitor Center. Except on holidays, you can obtain a map and information here and use the restrooms. If you want to explore the Arboretum, take a break from our route for that purpose now, or come back here later.

Our route proceeds through the Arboretum, along Meadow Road. Pass the maple tree area and come to the three picturesque ponds designed by Olmsted. Turn left into Forest Hills Road. Exit the Arboretum via the Forest Hills gate. Turn right along the Arborway and follow the road down the exit ramp to the Forest Hills T station.

Continuing on from the T station, cross Route 203 at the light. Here you find a sign welcoming you to the Pierre Lallement bicycle path. This path is dedicated in memory of the French gentleman who is attributed with "inventing the bicycle." (I sometimes fantasize what it might have been like to be a neighbor of someone inventing the bicycle, observing it from your window...)

The Pierre Lallement trail, also known as the Southwest Corridor Linear Park, follows the route of the T Orange Line above the ground right back to Back Bay. We are not going that far though. Take the trail past the first bridge over the T tracks then bear right into Williams Street past the English High School. Follow Williams Street one block to Washington Street where there is a special restaurant/pub destination.

F.J. Doyle's Braddock Café is one of the most famous eating and drinking places in Boston, and a worthy on-foot destination for anyone who enjoys food, beer, single-malt scotches, or just a great pub environment. Doyle's, which opened in 1882, has been a center of Irish political life back to the days of John F. Fitzgerald, the first Irish-American to become Mayor of Boston. It is frequented by such well-known folk as Senator John Kerry and Boston Mayor Tom Menino. There are photos celebrating visits by Bill Clinton and Senator Edward Kennedy (who dedicated the John F. Fitzgerald Room in memory of his late grandfather in 1988). Photos of Jack Kennedy and Franklin D. Roosevelt are also prominent. Breakfast is served every day, brunch is offered on Saturdays and Sundays, and you can expect a good time. One little caution: Doyle's does not accept credit cards.

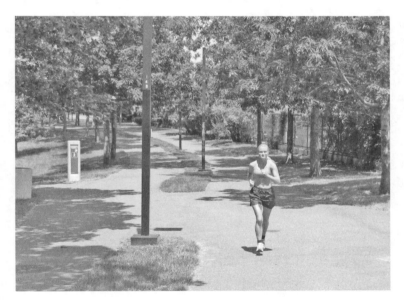

**The Lallement Trail near its Arboretum End**

After enough chatting with the locals at Doyle's, you can return to central Boston via the T Orange Line. Go back up Williams Street to the T line and Lallement trail, turn right along Amory Street, and find the Green Street T station two blocks further on.

If you are interested, the Samuel Adams Brewery is nearby and afternoon tours are offered some days of the week. To get to the brewery, continue north along the T line past Green Street a few short blocks to Porter Street. The brewery is in Porter Street. The Franklin Park Zoo is also within walking distance.

If you are still feeling energetic, you can take the Lallement trail on-foot back to Back Bay. We are disinclined to recommend that as it takes you near some more questionable parts of Boston, safety-wise. If you take that route, avoid straying east and south of the T line.

# South Boston Shore

| Distance | 7.9 miles |
|---|---|
| Comfort | Excellent on-foot conditions along an oceanfront trail for most of the route, with plenty of pedestrians around and few encounters with vehicle cross-traffic. The first half-mile and final mile-and-a-half are along street sidewalks. Crowds are unlikely to be a concern. Some parts are not suitable for inline skating. |
| Attractions | A beautiful ocean-side trail, passing popular beaches, the U. Mass. Campus, the JFK Library and Museum, and Castle Island/Fort Independence. Visit one of Boston's most famous residential areas, South Boston, with its Irish community. |
| Convenience | Start and end at T stations on the Red Line, which provides direct service to the financial district, downtown shops, theatre district, Cambridge, and southeastern Boston suburbs. Alternatively, you can easily walk from the end-point to the Seaport Hotel or the World Trade Center area. |
| Destination | Several excellent Irish pub/restaurants in South Boston. |

We now move to Boston's oceanfront routes. We start with a route in and around *Southie*, the number one residential area for Boston's Irish community. This route includes close to six miles of gorgeous oceanfront trails.

Take the T Red Line to the JFK/U Mass station and follow the signs "To Buses." Once outside, bear right and pass the bus area. There is a three-way road intersection here with a traffic signal. Pick up the street sidewalk of the rightmost road, heading south towards the supermarket. At the supermarket, take the footbridge over the road.

Continue south on the other side of the road, past the Boston College High School, to the main entrance road to the University of Massachusetts at Boston. Cross that road and pick up the paved pedestrian trail to the left, heading east along the waterfront. This is a very pleasant trail, far away from automobiles and with plenty of fresh ocean air. Continue to the JFK Library and Museum.

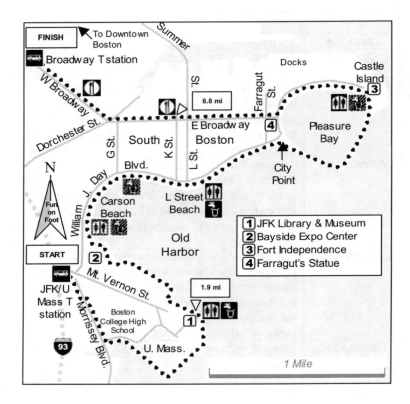

The JFK Library and Museum portrays the life and legacy of President Kennedy. Highlights include the family gallery of photographs and film coverage of the debate between John Kennedy and Richard Nixon in the 1960 presidential election campaign, the Cuban Missile Crisis, Walter Cronkite's announcement of the President's assassination, and the funeral. You probably do not want to interrupt your on-foot exercise at this early stage, but you might wish to come back here later.

Continue north and west on the coastal trail around the edge of the bay known variously as Old Harbor or Dorchester Bay. A short part of the trail is unsealed. On the opposite side of the bay is South Boston, your end destination. Just over a mile from the JFK library you come to Carson Beach, a popular local destination on hot summer days. From

that point on, follow beach frontage to City Point, where the beach ends
and a small collection of yacht clubs takes over the waterfront.

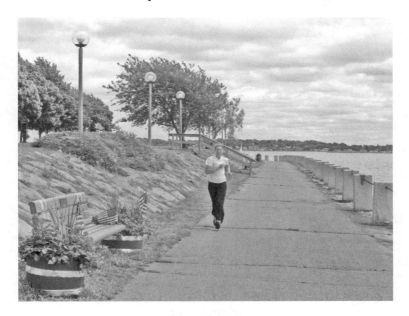

**The Ocean Trail by U. Mass.**

At this point you enter an interesting area known as Castle Island,
which comprises a large tidal pool (called Pleasure Bay), fully enclosed
by a manmade causeway. Go completely around the causeway (roughly
1.6 miles). If the wind is right, you might be entertained (or annoyed) by
low flying jet aircraft, landing or taking off at nearby Logan Airport.

At the northeast corner of the causeway you encounter Fort
Independence, on what was once a small island. This site has hosted
various forts since 1634, all known at their time as "The Castle." The
present edifice dates back to 1851 and played an active military role
right through World Wars I and II. Guided tours operate on Saturday
and Sunday afternoons, June through August, and Sundays in September
and October.

Continue following the paved trail from the fort, westward around
Pleasure Bay, until you encounter a statue of Admiral David Farragut
located somewhat haphazardly in the middle of the road. The U.S.
Navy's first admiral has stood here for over a hundred years, wistfully

scanning the horizon in vain for the first glimpse of a tall warship's topsails.

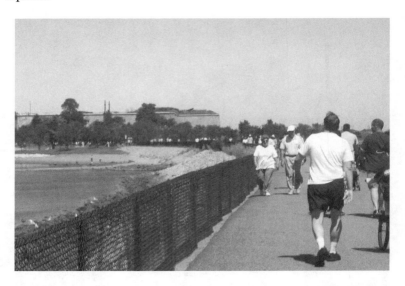

### The Pedestrian Causeway at Castle Island, Approaching Fort Independence

This statue and the Pleasure Bay causeway are all that remains of an 1890's vision to build a great Marine Park here, including a showcase aquarium. The South Boston Aquarium was built and did operate here from 1912 until 1954, when the whole venture tanked (pardon the pun) through lack of funds. The building was then razed. Now, this area contains a lovely beach, sporting, and recreation area—one of the best-kept locals' secrets.

Farragut's statue marks the eastern extremity of Broadway, the main thoroughfare threading South Boston end-to-end, and the road to follow to conclude this route.

South Boston is a famous and historical part of Boston, best known as the home of a large community of Irish immigrants. It follows that South Boston is also home to many Irish pubs, therefore an ideal place to end a nice day out on-foot.

The quality of South Boston's pubs varies widely. We like, in particular, the Playwright on E Broadway at K Street. It has a hearty atmosphere, a comprehensive food menu, and brunch on Saturday and Sunday. Running gear and non-locals are always welcome.

---

**VARIATION**

If you want to get back to the Seaport Hotel or World Trade Center area from near the Playwright, take L Street north from E Broadway. It leads straight to Summer Street in the middle of that part of the city.

---

Another good pub/restaurant choice is Shenannigans on W Broadway half a mile beyond the Playwright.

To get back to downtown Boston from either of these pubs, follow Broadway to the Broadway T station on the Red Line. The station is 1.1 miles from the Playwright.

Feel good about having touched the pulse of Boston's Irish heart!

# Quincy Shore and Neponset River

| | |
|---|---|
| **Distance** | 6.5 miles |
| **Comfort** | Roughly one mile is along regular street sidewalks. The rest is on dedicated pedestrian/bicycle trails either along the beachfront or off-street. Expect small numbers of other pedestrians or cyclists. Not suitable for inline skating in parts. |
| **Attractions** | A mix of excellent on-foot environments including paths through a natural park, along a marsh edge, along a 1.5-mile beachfront, and along a dedicated rail trail through the Neponset River Reserve. |
| **Convenience** | Start and end at stations on the T Red Line, roughly six miles southeast of downtown Boston. The Red Line provides direct service to the financial district, downtown shops, theatre district, Cambridge, and southeastern Boston suburbs. |
| **Destination** | The Lower Mills area on the Dorchester-Milton boundary. There are wind-down restaurant and bars here. |

We included this route because its on-foot conditions are second to none and it takes you through such a variety of different environments. It starts in Quincy, birthplace of John Hancock, John Adams, Howard Johnson's, and Dunkin Donuts. You traverse Merrymount Park, Quincy Shores, and Wollaston Beach. You then cross the Neponset River, and follow a new, dedicated rail-trail through the Neponset River Reserve.

Start at the T Red Line Wollaston station. Head north and east to the intersection of Hancock Street and Beale Street. Turn right into Hancock Street, pass Wollaston Avenue, and turn left into Merrymount Avenue. Follow Merrymount Avenue to its end, cross the street and go straight ahead to pick up the paved trail into Merrymount Park near the tennis courts.

Merrymount Park, with its wealth of natural forest, provides welcome escape from city and suburban life. Follow the paved trail to its end then take the gravel path to the north through the trees. It leads you to some sporting fields. Follow the road to the right to Merrymount Parkway, and turn left onto the parkway's sidewalk. Follow the sidewalk to the monument to John Adams and John Quincy Adams, father and son Presidents and two of this area's most famous citizens. Continue across the creek to Furnace Brook Parkway and turn left.

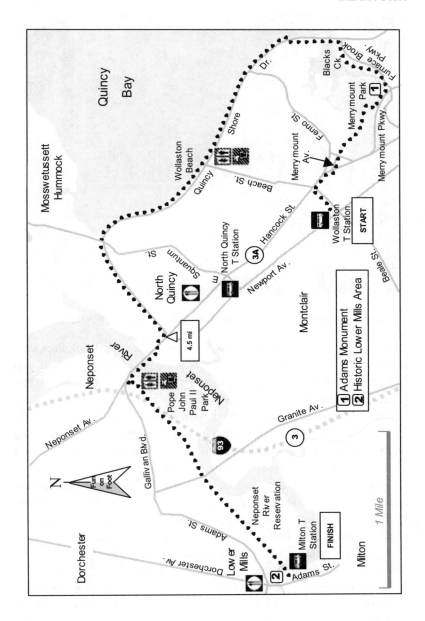

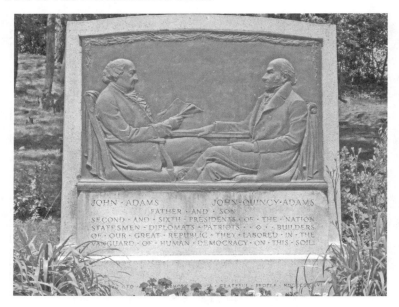

**Memorial to John Adams and John Quincy Adams**

Keep to the far left edge of the path along Furnace Brook Parkway. A dirt track peels off here and follows the edge of the marsh. If you like seeing marsh wildlife and getting away from all traffic, follow this track. Otherwise, use the street sidewalk.

After the track rejoins the street, you come to the intersection with Quincy Shores Drive. Turn left across the bridge and proceed to the picnic area and the pedestrian crossing light. Here you can safely cross Quincy Shores Drive to the beachfront sidewalk.

This is a very pleasant beach, with plenty of people on a nice day and views of the Boston skyline in the distance. There are restrooms at Elm Avenue, just before Beach Street. Keep following the beach roughly a mile and a half to its end at E Squantum Street.

Cross E Squantum Street and continue on Quincy Shore Drive. Where the road splits, keep to the right sidewalk and go down the ramp with the sign to the Quincy Business Area. Follow the ramp under the Neponset River road bridge. On the southern side of the bridge, climb the steps to the bridge walkway.

Cross the bridge. It is quite a pleasant crossing, with scenic views, although there is a lot of traffic close by. From the bridge you get to admire the new Pope John Paul II Park on the west side. At the end of bridge, double back along the street to the park. It is a very pleasant, grassy park with plenty of foot trails, sporting fields, a water fountain, and seasonal portable toilets.

You can circumnavigate the park, but it does not lead anywhere. We recommend bearing right to pick up the paved rail-trail.

The Granite Rail Corporation (1826-70) was the first incorporated railway company in the United States. It was built to transport granite from the Quincy Quarries to Gulliver's Creek Wharf on the Neponset River for building the Bunker Hill Monument. Now its rail-bed serves us on-footers admirably.

Follow the rail-trail to Granite Street. To cross Granite Street safely you need to divert up the street and cross at the light. The trail from here on is very shady and pleasant, and is joined by the light-rail line.

Continue to the Milton T station. Here you can catch a light rail car, which is logically an extension of the T Red Line, connecting at the Ashmont T station.

If you want a wind-down break first, climb the steps from the T station and turn right into the Lower Mills area of Dorchester.

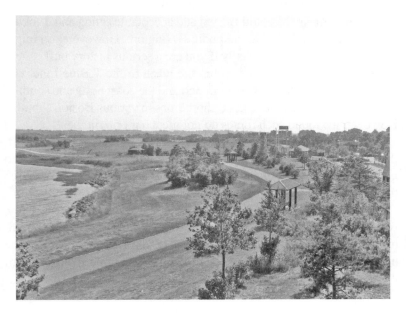

**Pope John Paul II Park**

Dorchester, established in 1630, was once the place containing the only powder-mill, paper-mill, and cracker, chocolate, and playing card factories in the nation. Lower Mills was the center of the milling activities into the mid-1900s. Today, plaques indicate the mill buildings that still stand.

There are a few acceptable eating and drinking joints around here. We enjoyed Donovan's Village Tavern and Restaurant in Dorchester Avenue, just north of Adams Street.

Be warned that parts of Dorchester have a somewhat shaky reputation today so, if you don't know the area, don't stray too far from here.


# Other Ideas

The **Minuteman Bikeway** is a paved cycling path that attracts some on-footers. It starts at the T Red Line Alewife station at Cambridge's western extremity and extends for 11 miles through historic Lexington (where the fighting of the American Revolution began in 1775), ending in Bedford. We did not document a route here because of the paucity of good return transit to central Boston and acceptable eating and drinking places at its logical turnaround point, Lexington. However, you might find it works for you, especially if you are a serious history buff.

North of downtown, and within the reach of the T Blue Line, you can find on-foot paths at **Revere Beach** and the coast north and south of there. There are also some good short loops in various Boston suburbs. However, we found such routes do not meet our criteria.

Further north along the coast, at **Nahant**, **Lynn**, and **Swampscott**, there are some excellent seaside trails of a good length. However, to get there you generally need to drive. There is a commuter rail service through this area, but it is not very frequent.

In **downtown** Boston, we have already covered what exists today. Note, however, that Boston is currently in the throes of a major facelift, in the wake of completion of the Big Dig and redevelopment of the harborfront area. We expect some nice shorter trails to result from that.

* * * *

One last piece of advice: Don't take it seriously when the Boston locals seem to be shunning all forms of communication with you, in particular, avoiding eye contact when you pass on a trail. New Englanders have a steely external reserve, but it does not go deep. Take the steps to open a communication channel and you will find a friendly and helpful person right there.

Enjoy Boston—site of the nation's conception! Now let's head south...

# 3

# The Big Apple

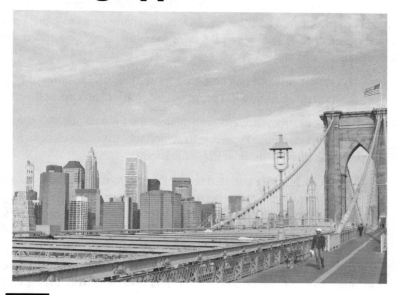

T hese vagabond shoes are longing to stray right through the very heart of it—New York, New York.[1]

This city oozes with history, entertainment, culture, fashion, and a unique rough-edges charm. There is everything you could ever want in a city—and, perhaps, a few other things too.

In central New York, on-foot is a very common means of transport. In fact, many Manhattan-dwellers don't own a car. Vehicles are enormously costly to operate and park, and not very efficient as a way to get around. The other option, the ad hoc combination of on-foot travel, public transit, and taxi, is frequently a better choice.

---

1   Julian Borger, lyricist.

Manhattan is very easy to navigate, at least above 14th Street, thanks to the grid system of numbered avenues and streets established in the visionary Commissioners' Plan of 1811. That simplifies life on the streets for city visitors. It does not, however, mean that driving is a breeze.

With New York's massive traffic volumes and narrow cross-town streets, driving is a challenge. Drivers are generally both very assertive and alert, and there is some synergy with Boston driving habits. However, some aspects of New York driving are very unique. What stands out most is the horn tooting. Over my many visits to New York I have researched the causes of the horn tooting. I have concluded the three main causes are:

- The driver in front has hesitated more than one hundredth of a second before hitting the pedal when a traffic gap appears;

- Some pedestrians are crossing against the light up ahead—this is actually a combined reaction in which the driver accelerates and blasts the horn solidly at the same time;

- The driver is very frustrated that nothing is moving and expresses such frustration via the horn. Since nothing moving is a very common state of affairs in New York traffic, you can easily appreciate that this one generates a lot of noise.

As a pedestrian though, be mindful of the second point. These drivers are a different breed to Boston drivers—a New York driver will happily plough through a pedestrian crossing at high speed with horns full a-blast, so do not bring any Boston-style pedestrian expectations here.

The other transport alternatives are the subway and the taxi.

The New York Subway system is one of the wonders of the modern world—unique in its kind. It provides good coverage of Manhattan, Brooklyn, the Bronx, and some parts of Queens. Its frequency is generally good. However, it has some strange behaviors. You can never know for sure exactly where a train will stop or what steps you might need to take to get to your final destination. The mystery is compounded by frequent PA announcements that are obviously trying to explain something but are totally unintelligible to everyone not wearing a Babel fish.[2]

One trip of ours was a classic. We had boarded a train from a Brooklyn extremity to Manhattan. However, as the trip progressed the stops became disconcertingly longer and the incomprehensible announcements more voluminous. Someone nearby (obviously wearing a Babel fish) advised that the announcements were saying there was a power failure on this line and the train would not be going much further. I pulled out my NYC Transit Map and started looking for alternative routes.

A friendly co-traveler intervened: "Forget the map. It won't help you!"

He was a local and was, of course, dead right. It turned out that the W-train we thought we were on was by now traveling on the N-train tracks as a result of a feat that my NYC Transit Map suggested was not even remotely possible. So don't take the map too seriously.

The best attitude is to simply find a train going in the general direction you want, such as Manhattan, and assume it will all work out in the end. In particular, do not worry. In our case, it effectively worked out. But this was only because we decided after two train changes (helped by the man with the Babel fish) to give up when we reached a Brooklyn station close to Manhattan where no trains were going in the right direction. (This was apparently due to more power failures.) We exited the subway and hailed a taxi to where we wanted to go.

This segues us to the other transport alternative—taxis. The New York taxi system has been very good for many years, and the only recent complaint is that it is starting to get as pricey as other cities. This is always a reasonable transport option, especially in Manhattan where taxis are plentiful, if your legs ever refuse to take you any further.

Running and jogging are quite popular in New York, although they are largely limited to a few popular parks or trails. In particular, it is simply not practical to run through the streets of Manhattan because of the many intersections encountered and the halts caused by the heavy vehicular and pedestrian traffic.

---

2        According to Douglas Adams, the *Hitchhiker's Guide to the Galaxy* explains how "if you stick a Babel fish in your ear you can instantly understand anything said to you in any form of language."

New York's climate, which is like Boston's but a touch warmer, is very good for on-foot exercise. The average daily maximum is in our preferred 40-to-80 degrees range every month except January, when it dips a little lower. There is precipitation on average 121 days of the year, so there is some risk of a shower dampening your day.

There are many excellent restaurants and pubs throughout New York that make for great food and beverage destinations. While some guidebooks still talk about the dress codes prevalent in New York, that dress code has almost entirely gone out the window now, except for high-end restaurants. There is no problem going into pubs or lower-end restaurants in running gear. Tourists, with their typical penchant for casual gear, have dictated this relaxation in attitude.

In New York today, street safety is not the big concern it once was. According to FBI statistics, New York's violent crime index (violent crimes per 1,000 residents in 2003) is 7.3, among the best for cities we cover. Certainly, I am amazed how safe it now feels in areas that I would not have ventured into alone 20 years ago. The city has done an amazing job of cleaning itself up. However, always use due street-sense and, in particular, avoid depressed or deserted areas.

The locals you meet in New York will unquestionably be a ton of fun. They all have, of course, that New York attitude; so do not expect to be treated like someone special. However, if you can handle that, you will love both the place and the people.

Even the New York pigeons have an attitude. This is the only place I know where the pigeons on the sidewalks will not get out of your way. After all, this is *their* city and—remember—you are not someone special!

We have put together a few routes that we believe will not fail to enthuse the city visitor or resident who likes on-foot action. We describe four routes that offer interesting environments and good running conditions in and close to Manhattan. We also describe two routes into the depths of Brooklyn for anyone feeling a little more adventurous and interested in exploring, at first hand, life in that highly cosmopolitan borough.

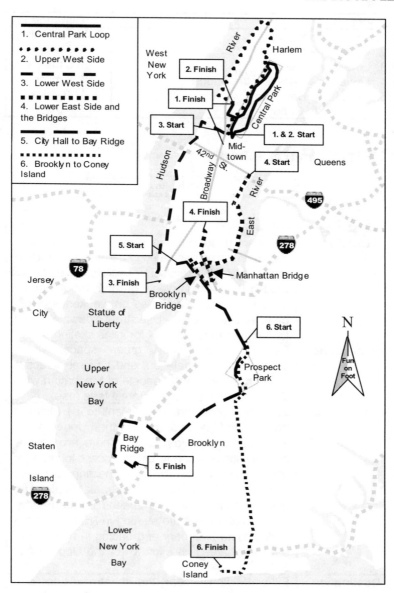

1. Central Park Loop
2. Upper West Side
3. Lower West Side
4. Lower East Side and the Bridges
5. City Hall to Bay Ridge
6. Brooklyn to Coney Island

West New York

River

Harlem

2. Finish

1. Finish

3. Start

1. & 2. Start

Central Park

Mid-town

42nd St.

4. Start

Queens

Hudson

Broadway

4. Finish

East River

495

278

5. Start

Jersey

78

3. Finish

Manhattan Bridge

City

Brooklyn Bridge

Statue of Liberty

6. Start

N

Fun on Foot

Upper New York Bay

Prospect Park

Staten

Bay Ridge

Brooklyn

Island

278

5. Finish

Lower New York Bay

6. Finish

Coney Island

**New York Routes**

| Route | Distance |
|---|---|
| 1. Central Park Loop | 5.9-to-6.4 miles |
| 2. Upper West Side | 7.7 miles |
| 3. Lower West Side | 6.0 miles |
| 4. Lower East Side and the Bridges | 7.8 miles |
| 5. City Hall to Bay Ridge | 11.9 miles |
| 6. Brooklyn to Coney Island | 8.0 miles |

# Central Park Loop

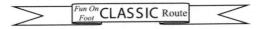

| | |
|---|---|
| **Distance** | 5.9-to-6.4 miles |
| **Comfort** | Excellent underfoot conditions in the park, on a path or in a lane dedicated to pedestrians. Expect many on-foot exercisers, cyclists, and others around but there is plenty of room for all. In the park, there are no vehicles on weekends or off-peak most weekdays. Use street sidewalks to get to and from the park. OK for inline skating. |
| **Attractions** | Beautifully landscaped green space, varied terrain, varied vegetation, and several attractive lakes. See where the people of Manhattan wind down. Various points of interest (see map). |
| **Convenience** | Start and finish are convenient to all Midtown hotels, and addresses on the Upper West Side and Upper East Side. There are several subway stations handy, giving access to all major north-south subway lines, connecting to Lower Manhattan, Brooklyn, and the Bronx. Stations for east-west subway lines to Queens are also nearby. We describe the route starting in Midtown at the park's south boundary and ending in a choice of restaurant areas, in Midtown or the Upper West Side. |
| **Destination** | Either Midtown near the theatre district and Times Square, or the Upper West Side. In both cases there are many excellent casual pubs and restaurants for winding down. |

While I have not found the statistics to prove it, I have no doubt that this is the most popular on-foot exercise route in the world. It is standard fare for locals and fitness-conscious visitors alike.

Central Park is a 2.5-mile by 0.5-mile tasteful nature preserve, bang in the middle of the densest population area of the country. It is easily reached on-foot from any hotel or residence in Midtown, the Upper West Side, or the Upper East Side.

Interestingly, Central Park was not a part of the Commissioners' Plan of 1811 that established the master street plan for Manhattan. Rather, it was the result of another stroke of planning brilliance in 1853, when both political parties at that time endorsed the idea of a large, central public park. Between 1853 and 1856 the city commissioners paid more than $5 million for undeveloped land from 59th Street to 106th Street, between Fifth and Eighth Avenues. The city commissioners then sponsored a public competition to design the new Central Park. Out of 33 anonymous entries they chose the "Greensward Plan," of Frederick Law Olmsted, the park superintendent, and local architect Calvert Vaux. Olmsted, born in Hartford Connecticut, subsequently became recognized as the father of American landscape architecture. Central Park was his first great work, to be followed later by several other major urban landscaping projects, including Boston's Emerald Necklace.

Central Park contains 58 miles of pedestrian paths, not all of which are suitable for running because of crowds of slow people in some parts. The most popular route is a 6.1-mile road circuit, Park Drive (also known as West Drive and East Drive on the respective sides of the park). This road is closed to vehicles on weekends year-round and in off-peak hours on weekdays except for the period from Thanksgiving through New Year. There is also a 1.6-mile jogging path around the reservoir. There are restrooms spread throughout the park, and ample other facilities such as food outlets and water.

Our nominal route simply follows the Park Drive loop, although you may want to deviate from that. When Park Drive is closed to vehicles, it is used by large numbers of on-foot exercisers, cyclists, inline skaters, and strolling pedestrians, but there is plenty of room for all. Even when it is open to vehicles, its side recreation path is fine for the on-foot exerciser.

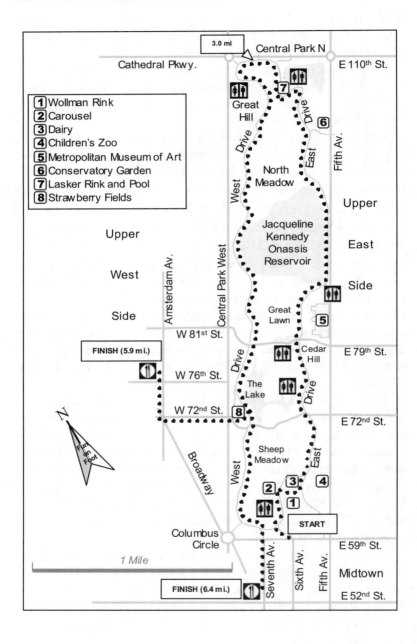

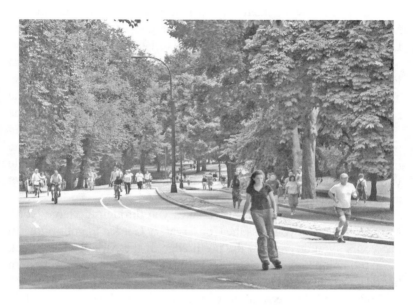

**Typical Weekend Scene on Park Drive**

The vehicular traffic (if any) and bicycle traffic travel counter-clockwise around the loop. Most pedestrians go that way too, although that is not essential and there is even a park recommendation that runners go the opposite direction. We shall assume counterclockwise for this route.

Our assumed start-point is at Central Park South, another name for 59th Street where it borders the park. There are park entrances at Sixth (Avenue of the Americas), Seventh, and Eighth Avenues. You can easily get here walking or running from any Midtown Hotel, or by riding any of several subway lines. For example, exit the subway at a 57th Street or Seventh Avenue/53rd Street Station.

Follow the road or path north a short distance until you reach Park Drive, then turn right. There are many things you may want to see in Central park, and we shall not mention all of them. One place you might want to swing by near the start of your route is the Dairy. It is down a path to the right off Park Drive, where you can see the 1908-vintage carousel on the left. The Dairy contains an information center where you can obtain a free detailed map of the park.

Continue following the road, which takes you past the Metropolitan Museum of Art. On the left you pass the Great Lawn, formerly the Lower Croton reservoir until it was filled in 1937.

You then come to the recently dedicated Jacqueline Kennedy Onassis Reservoir. For New York on-foot enthusiasts, this is an important place. There is a 1.6-mile, very popular soft surface jogging path around the reservoir. On this loop, you get beautiful views of Midtown from the north end. In May you are treated to an environment of flowering pink cherry trees. While we have not included this jogging path in the mileage of our route, you might well want to add on a loop of it while you are here. You can access the path from Park Drive at E 90th Street and other points around the reservoir.

After the reservoir, Park Drive takes you through the large North Meadow area, and you pass the Conservatory Garden to your right. In due course you arrive near the north edge of the park at 110th Street. Keep following Park Drive as it circles back southward near the western boundary of the park.

Follow Park Drive south to your exit point (or keep going and do another loop if you are in a 12-mile frame of mind).

We can suggest two nice exit points. The first is at W 72nd Street. This is near Strawberry Fields, the beautifully landscaped garden of international peace dedicated to the memory of John Lennon. You should walk through here if you have not been here before.

Nola and I happened to be running in Central Park the day after George Harrison's death and were somehow drawn to Strawberry Fields. It turned out we were far from alone—many, many of the Beatles' faithful made their way to the same place to pay their respects at a spontaneous, peaceful memorial for the loss of a second Beatle.

If you exit the park at W 72nd Street and are ready for lunch or a drink, you are close to an excellent West Side eating and drinking area. Head west two avenues to Amsterdam Avenue. There are many great choices around here—our favorite is Westside Brewing Co. at W 76th Street and Amsterdam. We shall discuss this subject further in the coverage of our next route.

The other obvious exit point is back at Central Park South where we started. From here, you have easy access to the many Midtown eating and drinking establishments between Times Square and Central Park. We are partial to Rosie O'Grady's on Seventh Avenue at 52nd Street. If you like Irish Pubs or old New York saloons (Rosie's claims to be both), go no further. The food at Rosie's is good and the atmosphere warm and friendly. However, if Rosie's is not your taste, you will have no difficulty finding another nice wind-down spot around here.

If you are into museums or art galleries, you might prefer to exit the park on the east side, around the Metropolitan Museum of Art, where such institutions are clustered. Good eating and drinking places are sparser around there, but if you go on to Third Avenue, you can find several good places from here on eastward.

# Upper West Side

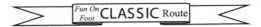

| Distance | 7.7 miles |
|---|---|
| Comfort | Good-to-excellent underfoot conditions with plenty of on-foot exercisers and cyclists around. Most of the route is on dedicated pedestrian/bicycle paths, but with a few blocks on street sidewalks. Not recommended overall for inline skating. |
| Attractions | Beautifully landscaped green space in Central Park and Morningside Park, then the natural beauty and interesting sights of Riverside Park and the Hudson. With a short diversion you can visit Grant's Memorial. |
| Convenience | Start and finish are convenient to all Midtown hotels and addresses on the Upper West Side. There are several subway stations handy, giving access to all major north-south subway lines, connecting to lower Manhattan, Brooklyn, and the Bronx. Stations for east-west subway lines to Queens are also nearby. We describe the route starting in Midtown at Central Park's south boundary and ending in a restaurant area on the Upper West Side. |
| Destination | Many excellent pubs and restaurants on the Upper West Side. |

While a loop of Central Park definitely has its appeal, we find this next route better overall. It includes Central Park as the northbound part of the route, but then switches over to the Hudson River and Riverside Park for the southbound return.

We suggest starting off with a three-mile half-loop of Central Park, taking you to the northwest corner of the park. While you could start from anywhere in the park, we shall assume starting from Central Park South in Midtown, as with our first route. This time, we shall assume following Park Drive in a clockwise direction, nearest the western boundary of the park, but you can choose a different route through Central Park if you wish.

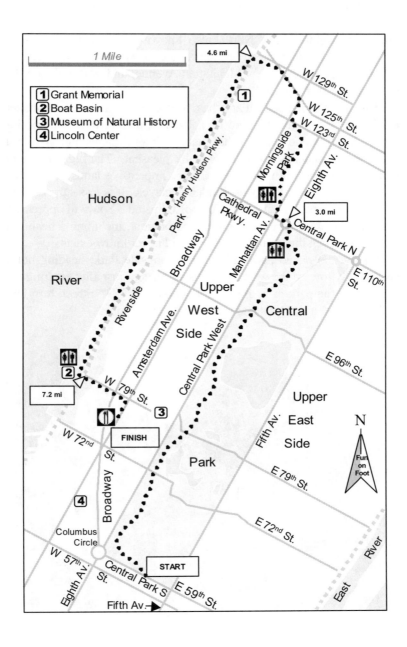

1 Mile

1 Grant Memorial
2 Boat Basin
3 Museum of Natural History
4 Lincoln Center

4.6 mi

W 129th St.
W 125th St.
W 123rd St.

Hudson

Henry Hudson Pkwy.

Morningside Park

Eighth Av.

Cathedral Pkwy.

Manhattan Av.

3.0 mi

Central Park N

River

Riverside

Broadway

Upper

Central

E 110th St.

West

Amsterdam Ave.

Central Park West

E 96th St.

Side

7.2 mi

W 79th St.

Fifth Av.

Upper

East

N

3

Side

Fun on Foot

FINISH

Park

E 79th St.

W 72nd St.

4

Broadway

E 72nd St.

Columbus Circle

River

W 57th St.

Central Park S

START

East

Eighth Av.

E 59th St.

Fifth Av.

Exiting Central park at its northwest corner brings you out on the streets at the intersection of Eighth Avenue and W 110th Street, also known as Central Park North, also known as Cathedral Parkway. Cross both streets and head one short block west on W 110th Street to Manhattan Avenue. Cross Manhattan Avenue, and you will find the entrance to Morningside Park.

30-acre Morningside Park has a decidedly different character to Central Park—much more of a locals' precinct than a place for everyone. In some respects that makes it more interesting. While it is not immaculately kept, it is generally pleasant. The big surprise in store in Morningside Park is some very impressive landscaping, that can rival Central Park's nicest hidden enclaves. It is less surprising to learn that this park is also the work of Olmsted. You will appreciate passing through a very impressive environment, including a beautiful waterfall, which the average tourist would never know exists.

Follow the paved path through Morningside Park, heading north and slightly toward the west. There is a restroom just after entering the park. Exit the park at its northern boundary, W123rd Street, turn left, and head west a short distance to Amsterdam Avenue.

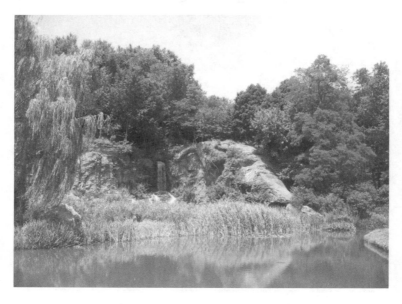

**The Hidden Beauty of Morningside Park**

There are various ways from here to the Hudson River. All require traversing very ordinary streets for a few blocks.

We suggest going two short blocks up Amsterdam Avenue to W 125th Street and then follow that street to the left to its intersection with W 129th Street. (Alternatively, cut through the Morningside Gardens apartment complex to La Salle Street and Broadway, then take Broadway northward to W 125th Street.) Once on W 129th Street, take the underpass under the Henry Hudson Parkway to pick up the Hudson River Promenade.

---

**VARIATION**

Here is an alternative route to the river, starting from W 123rd Street and Amsterdam Avenue. It has the disadvantage of poorer underfoot terrain, including some hills, but it has some attractions of its own. Head westward up the hill on W 123rd Street. It will bring you to the tomb of Ulysses S. Grant, victorious Union commander in the Civil War and two-term President. Grant's tomb hides up on the bluffs above the river, in a granite and marble structure a little reminiscent of the Jefferson Memorial in Washington, DC. It remains the largest mausoleum in North America today. If you trek up here, to get back to our main route you will then need to work your way north to W 125th Street to gain access to the Hudson River Promenade. Alternatively, head south and pick up the Riverside Park pedestrian trail along the top of the bluffs. You will later find linking paths down to the Promenade.

---

Riverside Park is a 323-acre park adjacent to the Hudson River from 68th to 155th Street. This park was developed initially in the latter quarter of the nineteenth century and has been extended since. It includes sculptures and memorials exalting several of the city's heroes, plus many recreational facilities. Most importantly, it has excellent trails for on-foot exercise, with pleasant scenery all round.

There are trails at two different levels. The first is the Promenade, which follows the riverbank the entire length of the park (except possibly for interruptions due to construction or maintenance). You are immediately adjacent to the water with views of the New Jersey side opposite. The second trail, which is wider but not quite so visually interesting, is inside the Henry Hudson Parkway. Below 104th Street you can find various paths to switch between these trails.

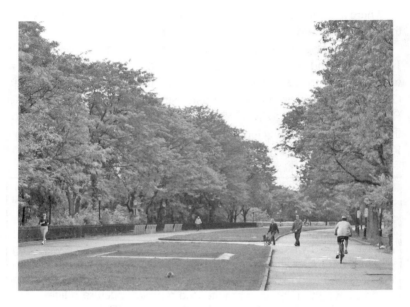

**The Spacious Main Pedestrian and Cyclist Trail in Riverside Park**

Assuming you take the Promenade, continue all the way down to W 79th Street. There you will encounter the 79th Street Boat Basin and the Boat Basin Café. Depending on the time of year and the weather, you might find this a very pleasant spot to relax and lunch. (It is not necessarily open every day.) If it is open, the food is ordinary but the atmosphere on a lovely day compensates for any culinary deficiencies.

If you want to keep following Riverside Park further, you can continue down to W 72nd Street or its end at W 68th Street, then head left back to the theatre district. South of 68th Street, a bicycle trail continues on to link up with the lower Hudson trail (see our next route). However, the next stretch is through a docks area and is less pleasant than what you have experienced in this route so far.

For our favored route, we suggest you exit Riverside Park at W 79th Street and head two or three blocks east to Broadway or Amsterdam Avenue in the heart of the Upper West Side dining area. Here you will find many choices for eating, drinking, or both. You will unquestionably find a satisfying destination here.

We have sampled several places around here. If pressed for a recommendation, Nola's and mine would be Westside Brewing Co. at 76th Street and Amsterdam. While not actually a brewery any more, it offers a good selection of beers, a comprehensive and reasonable quality food menu, Saturday and Sunday Brunch, and lots of good company and cheer all around.

Nola and I had one particularly memorable afternoon at Westside Brewing. We just happened to be there in 2003, watching an American League baseball finals game between the Red Sox and the Yankees. It turned out to be a very violent and controversial game, with bench-clearing brawls and considerable physical violence between players, staff, and others. At Westside Brewing, we Red Sox fans were, not surprisingly, far outnumbered by Yankees fans. There was much loud debate amongst everyone in the establishment throughout the on-field debacle. However, we all ended up laughing and drinking together in cheery spirits. This is a glowing commendation for a good company pub for all-comers.

After winding down from your on-foot exercise at a good establishment around here, you can easily walk back to your Midtown hotel or brave the NYC subway to take you to other transit destinations.

# Lower West Side

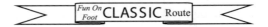

| Distance | 6.0 miles |
|---|---|
| **Comfort** | Excellent underfoot conditions throughout on mostly dedicated pedestrian trails. No vehicle concerns. Expect plenty of other people about. OK for inline skating. |
| **Attractions** | Innumerable cultural and recreational activities throughout, plus scenic views of the lower Hudson and the Statue of Liberty. Specific attractions include the Intrepid Sea, Air, and Space Museum, Hudson River Park, the Irish Hunger Memorial, Museum of Jewish Heritage, the World Trade Center Sphere and eternal flame, and historic Castle Clinton. |
| **Convenience** | Start at Columbus Circle in Midtown, handy to hotels and several subway lines. End in lower Manhattan with convenient subway access back to Midtown. |
| **Destination** | Battery Park and the Financial District, with many attractions and many excellent eating/drinking establishments for winding-down. |

If you are familiar with the lower west side of the past, with its row upon row of run-down docks and grimy industrial sites, you might be in for a surprise with this next route. Over the past few years this part of Manhattan has been largely transformed into a pleasant recreational area, thanks mainly to these initiatives: Hudson River Park, Battery Park City Parks Conservancy, and the Battery Conservancy, respectively.

When complete, Hudson River Park will be a 550-acre park stretching from W 59th Street down to the south end of Manhattan. When we were last there, work was still in progress, but we have no hesitation in declaring this a very enjoyable on-foot route today.

You can start out from anywhere in Midtown by heading west to the Hudson River bank. We nominally start at Columbus Circle at the southwest corner of Central Park, a spot that is easily reached from various subway lines or on-foot from most midtown hotels. From the

Circle, head west along W 58th Street to Twelfth Avenue, cross that street, and pick up the paved trail heading south.

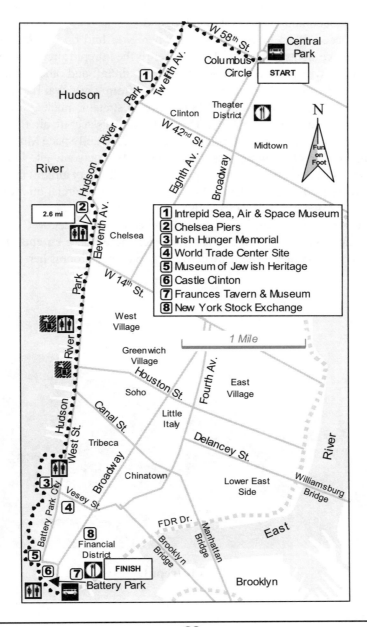

While the trail is sometimes shared with cyclists, progressively more pedestrian-dedicated parts are being built. The most northerly part is the least attractive, with considerable noisy traffic nearby. However, underfoot conditions are consistently good.

Proceed down to W 46th Street, where you find one of the most impressive sights of any city. Docked here is the Intrepid aircraft carrier, complete with a large collection of historic aircraft and other military relics on its deck. The Intrepid was in service from World War II through to 1974. Alongside it is the USS Growler, a strategic nuclear missile submarine (open to the public). This collection of sea craft, aircraft and other memorabilia, known as the Intrepid Sea, Air and Space Museum, is rounded out by nothing less than a Concorde supersonic jet. In fact, it is not just any Concorde, but Concorde AD—the very aircraft that set the record for fastest Atlantic crossing by any commercial aircraft (2 hours, 52 minutes, and 59 seconds).

Continue southward, past the heliport at W 30th Street, to Chelsea Piers around W 20th Street. The four piers here house an enormous recreation complex. There are convenient public restrooms here.

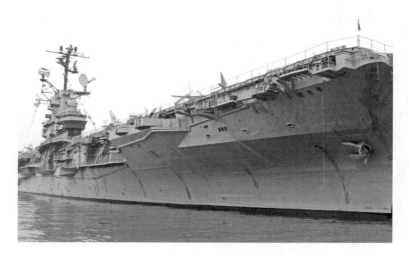

**USS Intrepid**

**VARIATION**
If you want to see the Intrepid Museum, one suggestion is to do this route in reverse, starting out from Battery Park (the southern end of the No. 1 subway line) and making this museum your destination. After exploring the museum, then simply head east to wind-down at one of the many restaurants in and north of the theater district, around Seventh or Eighth Avenue.

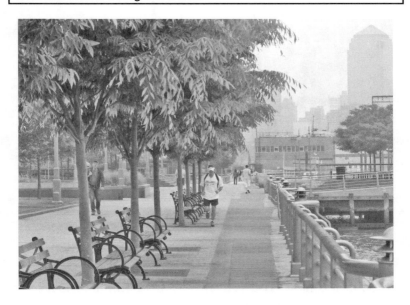

**Hudson River Park**

As you approach the Greenwich Village part of the park, make sure to use the pedestrian-only trail right on the riverfront, rather than the bike trail. By the time you get to Pier 45, around W 10th Street, conditions have become excellent for the on-foot exerciser. The traffic is now well away, and the landscaping and views are very attractive. Pier 45 and the esplanade between it and Pier 46 are one of the first parts of Hudson River Park to be fully developed. It is pleasant and relaxing, with grass and shade areas, restrooms, and concessions.

At Pier 40 near Houston Street, there is another pleasant recreation area, with various sporting facilities. Houston (pronounced *how-stun*, unlike that great city in the South) is the east-west street in Lower Manhattan that marks the end of the numbered street system. After

Houston you get to see the Trapeze School of New York at work, flying through the air. Then, at Pier 25 near N Moore Street, you find the Children's Park and the Hudson River Sculpture Garden.

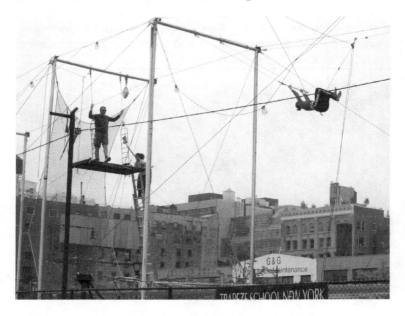

**The Trapeze School of New York**

You then come to Battery Park City, a modern development on the lower Hudson comprising a tasteful combination of residences, businesses, and recreational spaces. Battery Park City is an excellent area for the on-footer, with the Statue of Liberty always in sight. First you take a sharp right to follow the river's edge. Continue to where you are forced to do a sharp left, around the edge of Governor Nelson A. Rockefeller Park with its large grassed area. At Vesey Street, you pass the Irish Hunger Memorial, remembering the 1845-49 Irish potato famine, when blight destroyed the Irish potato crop. Deprived of their staple food, over a million Irish died.

Continue past the North Cove Yacht Harbor, the Esplanade where many community sports and other recreational activities are available, then lantern-decorated South Cove. There are also some restaurants and bars around here. Pass the Museum of Jewish Heritage and Robert

F. Wagner Jr. Park before leaving Battery Park City and entering historic Battery Park proper, the end destination of our route.

In Battery Park there are various attractions including Pier A, the last remaining example of Victorian waterfront architecture in New York; Castle Clinton, an 1811 fort built to defend New York Harbor; and the World Trade Center Sphere and an eternal flame, memorializing the lives lost on 9/11. The Sphere was retrieved from the ruins of the World Trade Center. This is also where crowds line up to visit the Statue of Liberty.

At this point you are also handy to the Financial District, and you can easily walk north to the World Trade Center site or northeast to the New York Stock Exchange, should you wish to visit such places.

There are many places to wind-down for some food and beverage around here. For a wide selection of food that you can consume in an outdoor seating area, there is the Amish Market at 17 Battery Place, just out of Battery Park. If you are more interested in a restaurant/ pub, there are several excellent places in the financial district. Most notable is Fraunces Tavern & Museum, a short walk northeast of the park at 54 Pearl Street. Built in 1719, it is best known as the site where Washington bade farewell to the officers of the Continental Army in 1783. There is a casual bar area, as well as a more up-market restaurant. We can also recommend the cozy Ulysses Irish Pub at 95 Pearl Street or Pound and Pence at 55 Liberty Street.

To take a subway back to Midtown, there are various options. The simplest is the No. 1 train, which leaves from the station at the bottom end of Battery Park and will drop you virtually anywhere the length of Broadway.

# Lower East Side and the Bridges

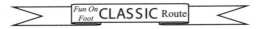

| | |
|---|---|
| **Distance** | 7.8 miles |
| **Comfort** | Good-to-excellent underfoot conditions with plenty of on-foot exercisers and cyclists around. 70% of the route is on dedicated pedestrian or pedestrian/bicycle paths; the rest is on street sidewalks. Not recommended for inline skating. |
| **Attractions** | The fresh air of the East River and the unforgettable panoramic views of Manhattan crossing both the Brooklyn Bridge and the Manhattan Bridge. |
| **Convenience** | Start on the east side of Midtown, at the United Nations Building (E 42$^{nd}$ Street) or as far south as E 25$^{th}$ Street. You can easily get here on foot from any Midtown hotel or Grand Central station where the No. 4, 5, 6, and 7 subways stop. End in Houston Street in central Lower Manhattan. You can walk to Midtown or the financial district from there, or take a subway. |
| **Destination** | The focus point for innumerable excellent pubs and restaurants in Chinatown, Little Italy, Soho, and Greenwich Village. Lower Manhattan tourist destinations such as Washington Square, the Financial District, and Battery Park are nearby. |

If you have never crossed the Brooklyn Bridge on foot, you have missed out on one of life's great experiences. There lies one of several compelling reasons to try this next route.

Our previous two routes followed the Hudson River. Manhattan's other river, the East River, also has a bicycle and pedestrian path most of its length, except for a large annoying gap in Midtown. We shall restrict our coverage of this river to the lower part, which is the most appealing. This trail, while it does not offer much in the way of big-city-escape, does offer impressive sights of massive skyscrapers and bridges and also the opportunity to cross some of those bridges for some unforgettably spectacular views. If you have not done this route before, it is a must-do!

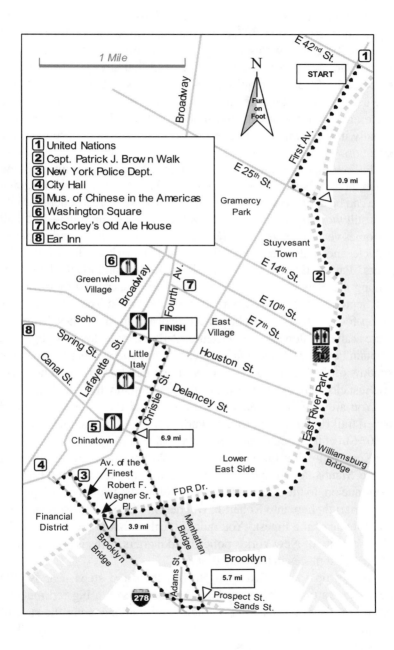

1 Mile

N
Fun
on
Foot

START

**1** United Nations
**2** Capt. Patrick J. Brown Walk
**3** New York Police Dept.
**4** City Hall
**5** Mus. of Chinese in the Americas
**6** Washington Square
**7** McSorley's Old Ale House
**8** Ear Inn

E 42nd St.

**1**

First Av.

Broadway

E 25th St.

0.9 mi

Gramercy
Park

Stuyvesant
Town

E 14th St.

**2**

**6**

Greenwich
Village

Broadway

Fourth Av.

**7**

E 10th St.

E 7th St.

Soho

East
Village

**FINISH**

Houston St.

**8**

Spring St.

Lafayette St.

Little
Italy

Delancey St.

Canal St.

Christie St.

**5**

Chinatown

6.9 mi

Lower
East Side

East River Park

Williamsburg
Bridge

**4**

Av. of the
Finest
Robert F.
Wagner Sr.
Pl.

**3**

FDR Dr.

Financial
District

3.9 mi

Brooklyn
Bridge

Manhattan
Bridge

Brooklyn

278

Adams St.

5.7 mi

Prospect St.
Sands St.

We nominally start at the United Nations Headquarters at E 42nd Street and First Avenue. In fact, you can start anywhere on First Avenue above E 25th Street, without losing any of this route's value. The reason is the Midtown gap in the East River trail that stretches from E 63rd Street to E 25th Street, requiring on-foot exercisers to use the sidewalk of First Avenue for this stretch. However, this is not really so bad, since there are few cross streets and modest traffic volume. You are also usually in the company of other on-foot exercisers who face the same situation.

Follow First Avenue to E 25th Street, where you can turn left and reach the riverbank. Then turn right, heading downstream. The going here can be a little confusing initially—when we were last here the city was still working on fixing the bicycle and pedestrian trails—but it all becomes very organized by E 18th Street. There, a clearly marked paved bicycle and pedestrian trail—the Captain Patrick J. Brown Walk—starts. Patrick Brown, a renowned local military and FDNY hero, was among the New York firefighters that bravely sacrificed their lives in the September 11, 2001 destruction of the World Trade Center. As an on-foot exerciser himself, in accordance with his wishes, his ashes were scattered along a trail in Central Park where he loved to jog. The Captain Patrick J. Brown Walk is such a fitting memorial, passing in the shadow of the Stuyvesant Town apartment building in which he lived, and just close enough to the site of the building in which he died.

You are now in the area called East River Park. There is a good paved trail right down to Battery Park at Manhattan's southern tip. At E 10th Street there are restrooms and a water fountain.

Keep following the trail under the Williamsburg Bridge then on to the Manhattan Bridge. There are excellent views of the bridges. Continue on, to the street immediately before the Brooklyn Bridge.

Turn right here into Robert F. Wagner Sr. Place. This leads you into the Avenue of the Finest. You quickly realize that you are now in the close vicinity of New York's police headquarters. This is probably one of the safest places in the United States.

To get up to the Brooklyn Bridge, there are steps near NYPD headquarters that take you up to a concourse with a big red metallic sculpture. Bear left past the sculpture and you encounter the start of the pedestrian path onto the Brooklyn Bridge. While this may all be a bit confusing, never fear since there are always many police officers around here who can direct you. (Nola and I needed to use exactly that service the first time here.)

Running (or walking) the Brooklyn Bridge is an unforgettable experience.

This bridge, now a National Historic Landmark, was opened in 1883. The intrigue surrounding the Brooklyn Bridge started with its enthusiastic designer, John A. Roebling, dying as a result of an accident during its construction and failing to ever see the result. For pedestrians and cyclists, the bridge is outstanding. Rather than using a sidewalk near a busy roadway, which is the case in every other bridge I know, pedestrians and cyclists are treated to a nice elevated pathway, amongst the cables high above the traffic. This not only keeps the traffic noise reasonable but also opens up panoramic views of New York City for the entire crossing. You typically encounter many other pedestrians and some cyclists, but are unlikely to experience sufficiently large crowds to be a problem.

At the Brooklyn end of the bridge, the path splits. Follow the left-hand, lower path, which takes you to the streets below the bridge. You are about to skirt the area known as Dumbo—from "Down Under the Manhattan Bridge Overpass." I kid you not—New York really has the most creative precinct names of anywhere I know! Follow Prospect Street westward, turn right at Adams Street, and then turn left into Sands Street. This takes you to the Manhattan Bridge. There are signs here to the bicycle and pedestrian walkways. The southern walkway is now dedicated to pedestrians only, the northern one being for cyclists only. You have excellent views of the Financial District buildings and the Brooklyn Bridge from the pedestrian walkway. (Once again pedestrians win out over cyclists!) The main problem with this bridge is the noise from not only the vehicle traffic but also the trains that use the bridge. Nevertheless, you will unquestionably be glad you experienced it.

The pedestrian walkway exits in the middle of Chinatown, so if you are ready for a Chinese meal your route has ended. However, there are also many other interesting restaurant areas within a short walk or jog of here. They include (moving progressively northward) Little Italy, Soho, and Greenwich Village. There are, in fact, way too many restaurants and bars around here for anyone to classify and compare them all.

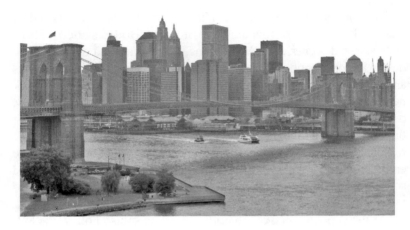

## The View from the Manhattan Bridge

After much thought we decided to lead you to roughly the nucleus of this eating and drinking zone, which happens to be at our favorite Irish pub/restaurant in these parts, Puck Fair. This fine establishment is at the intersection of Houston and Lafayette Streets, in Soho. Soho, by the way, means "south of Houston." Washington Square, Greenwich Village, East Village, and Little Italy are all a hop and a skip from here.

To get to Puck Fair from the Manhattan Bridge, first go one block east to Christie Street; follow relatively sedate Christie Street north to Houston Street; then turn left and head west a few blocks on Houston to Lafayette Street. Puck Fair is a top-class Irish Pub with excellent food, décor, and atmosphere. Its name reflects a pre-Celtic pagan festival still held in Killorglin, County Kerry, in August every year. The festival focuses around a goat theme.

There are also some very historic drinking establishments not far from here, if you like that sort of thing. A little northeast of Puck Fair, on 7th Street, is McSorley's Old Ale House, founded in 1854 and totally unchanged since, right down to the sawdust on the floor. The food is not the best by today's standards, but the place sure has character. Also, further west in Spring Street is the historic Ear Inn, built in 1817, and a renowned pub (or speakeasy) for sailors most of its life. The name "Ear" was adopted when the "Bar" neon sign partly burned out.

If you want to see the tourist sights of Lower Manhattan, such as Wall Street, Battery Park, or the World Trade Center site, all of these are an easy walking distance away.

There are many subway stations throughout this area if you want to brave the subway system to get to your final destination. Alternatively, if Midtown is your destination and you have half an hour to spare, you can easily walk up there passing the Empire State Building on the way.

# City Hall to Bay Ridge

| | |
|---|---|
| **Distance** | 11.9 miles |
| **Comfort** | Moderate-to-excellent running conditions. Roughly 50% of the route is on dedicated pedestrian or pedestrian/bicycle paths; the rest is on street sidewalks. Expect some other pedestrians around for the entire route. Crowds are unlikely to be a problem except possibly in Downtown Brooklyn. Not recommended for inline skating because of the extensive use of street sidewalks. |
| **Attractions** | Cross the unforgettable Brooklyn Bridge, pass through Prospect Park, Brooklyn's answer to Central Park, experience the beauty of the Brooklyn shoreline, and touch the pulse of the diverse Brooklyn community. End in a lively Brooklyn precinct in the shadows of the Verrazano-Narrows Bridge. |
| **Convenience** | Start in Lower Manhattan and end in the lively Brooklyn neighborhood of Bay Ridge. There are several subway stations handy to the start. From the end-point, you can catch the R-train to Downtown Brooklyn, Lower Manhattan, Midtown, or Queens. |
| **Destination** | Several excellent pubs and restaurants in the Bay Ridge region of Brooklyn. |

Manhattan is just one of five boroughs comprising New York City—Brooklyn, Queens, Bronx, and Staten Island are the others. Having covered the best of Manhattan, we felt compelled to also seek routes in Brooklyn, which has the attraction of a long shoreline and is particularly handy to Manhattan via bridge and subway.

Brooklyn, home to almost 2.5 million people, has a history stretching back to 1646. In that year, the Village of Breuckelen was created by the Dutch West India Company and became the first municipality in what is now New York State (Albany and New York followed). In 1683, after the British had taken over, Kings County was established here, along with eleven other counties forming the province of New York. Brooklyn was one town in Kings. All of the pieces of Kings County were subsequently absorbed into the one City of Brooklyn. In 1898, that city merged with the City of New York, which before that time had only included Manhattan and the Bronx.

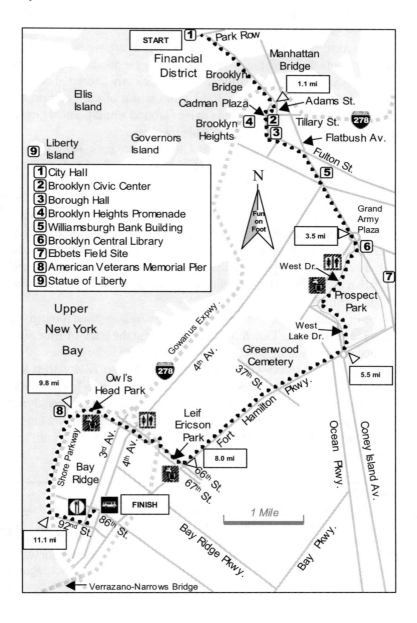

From its origins until today, Brooklyn has been the chosen place for settling by a wide variety of different cultural and ethnic groups. The resultant blend of diverse cultural sub-communities makes Brooklyn a place of tremendous character.

Since most New York visitors stay in Manhattan, we start our first Brooklyn route there. This also gives the on-footer another opportunity to experience the Brooklyn Bridge. We have clearly exceeded our 10-mile upper limit on this route. If 12 miles is out of the question for you, you can easily break the route in half around a mid-point at Grand Army Plaza or Prospect Park, reachable by subway.

We nominally start the route at City Hall in Park Row, Lower Manhattan. This point is close to several subway stations and is a short walk from hotels in the Financial District.

Starting from City Hall, head east along Park Row and pick up the pedestrian ramp onto the Brooklyn Bridge. Ask a local if you have trouble finding it. As described in our prior route, crossing the Brooklyn Bridge on foot is an experience not to be missed. This time though, after crossing the bridge, take the right hand (upper) path where the pedestrian trail splits. This will head you towards Downtown Brooklyn on Adams Street.

You have different options now. The following suggested route gives you some exposure to Downtown Brooklyn and the edge of Brooklyn Heights, without adding much distance to shorter possible routes.

Where Adams meets Tillary Street, turn right into Tillary, then left into Cadman Plaza. Pass Brooklyn Civic Center and turn left at Fulton Street (or Joralemon Street). This will take you past one of Brooklyn's most architecturally interesting buildings—the Borough Hall, a Greek revival building built in 1849. It served as Brooklyn City Hall until fire damaged much of it in 1895.

---

**VARIATION**

If you do not mind adding a mile and a couple of hills, you can take in the panoramic sights a few blocks west of Cadman Plaza at Brooklyn Heights Promenade. From Tillary, turn right into Cadman Plaza then left into Clark Street and follow it to its end. Work your way south to Montague Street, enjoy the views, and then follow Montague to the Civic Center.

---

Continue along Fulton Street, which becomes Fulton Mall, a central shopping area. The going here is not the best but you certainly will have the opportunity to experience the feel of Downtown Brooklyn at first hand.

Keep following Fulton Street to Flatbush Avenue, and turn right there. Head towards the Williamsburgh Bank Building, Brooklyn's tallest structure. At this point, if you are wondering why we led you to such an ordinary, unbeautiful urban area, fear not since conditions will soon improve significantly.

---

**VARIATION**
You can cut 0.3 mile off the route as follows. From Adams Street turn left into Tillary Street then right into Flatbush Avenue. This variation bypasses Downtown Brooklyn but takes you through a quite drab and uninteresting quarter.

---

Follow Flatbush Avenue south to Grand Army Plaza. Grand Army Plaza heralds the start of Prospect Park—Brooklyn's answer to Central Park. Olmsted and Calvert designed Prospect Park and the plaza as their encore to building Central Park. The planning started in 1860. After the project was interrupted by the Civil War, the park was completed for opening in 1868.

Grand Army Plaza, which was originally decorated with just a simple fountain, is dominated today by the Soldiers and Sailors Memorial Arch. The arch, styled somewhat like the Arc de Triomphe in Paris, was designed by John H. Duncan, who also designed Grant's Tomb in Manhattan. The arch was completed in 1896. The plaza now also contains a monument to John F. Kennedy and several other statues. The centerpiece Bailey Fountain, build in 1932 and recently restored, is a favorite backdrop in wedding portraits. A green market is held every Saturday, attracting many locals.

After passing through the plaza, you enter Prospect Park proper, with the stately Brooklyn Central Library to the left of the entrance. At 526 acres, Prospect Park is roughly two-thirds the size of Central park, and no less attractive. The park fell into a bad state of disrepair in the middle part of the twentieth century but, thanks to the Prospect Park Alliance, it is now well on its way back to the place of beauty originally envisaged by Olmsted and Vaux.

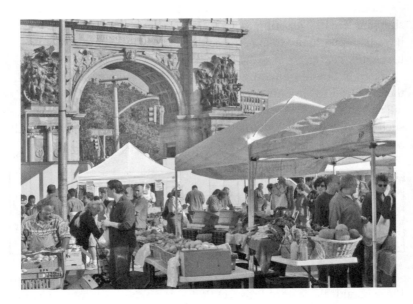

**Grand Army Plaza Memorial Arch and Green Market**

Similar to Central Park, Prospect Park has an internal roadway loop through it—3.3 miles around in this case. On the west side of the park it is variously called West Drive or West Lake Drive, and the names on the east side correspond. The roadway is usually closed to vehicles when on-foot exercisers want to be there; that is, on all weekends and in non-peak hours on weekdays in February through November. The consequence is beautiful on-foot exercise conditions. There are also many other pedestrian paths through the park, which you might wish to explore.

We suggest following West Drive, that is, bear right after entering the park. One of the park's most important features is on your left—the Long Meadow, a 60-acre expanse of green grass that lays claim to being New York's largest open green space.

There are various other points of interest along the route but, most importantly, Prospect Park is a locals' place for on-foot exercise and escape from the urban ruckus.

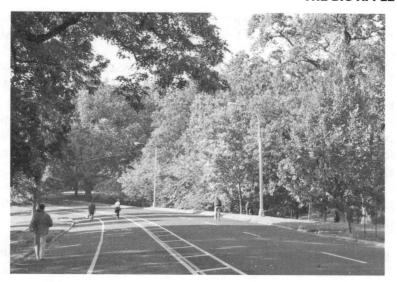

**Vehicle-Free West Drive in Prospect Park**

---

**VARIATION**
   If you were to go a short block beyond Prospect Park's eastern boundary at Montgomery Street, you would be where legendary Ebbets Field once stood.  This was home to the Brooklyn Dodgers from 1913 to 1957, prior to their transplanting to California.  Unfortunately, it is probably not worth the trip today, since just a plaque and apartment complexes fill the void resulting from the famous stadium's demolition in 1960.  However, it helps to be knowing and respectful with the locals on this sensitive topic.

---

   After West Drive becomes West Lake Drive, you pass the large and attractive Prospect Park Lake.  At the southernmost point in the park, two miles from where you entered Grand Army Plaza, a park exit takes you to a large rotary.  Follow the signs to Fort Hamilton Parkway, and take the right-hand sidewalk of that street.

   You now face 2.5 miles on this sidewalk.  The good news is that Fort Hamilton Parkway is a parkway—which in New York systematically means that no heavy trucks are allowed.  Furthermore, the sidewalk is wide and mostly uncrowded.  The bad news is that the car traffic can

---

be quite heavy. The enjoyment in this part of the route lies more in experiencing the variety of traditional life in Brooklyn than in any sort of scenic beauty.

After a few blocks, you reach the Greenwood Cemetery. Follow its southern edge to 37th Street. On-foot conditions in this part are very good, with no cross-street traffic.

The remaining 1.5 miles along Fort Hamilton Parkway, while not beautiful, illustrate Brooklyn's makeup very well. You traverse at least four distinct cultural sub-zones—eclectic, traditional Jewish, Chinese, and Middle Eastern. This is what characterizes Brooklyn!

The natural beauty re-emerges at 66th Street. Turn right into Leif Ericson Park, which occupies the land between 66th and 67th Streets most of the way to the shoreline.

Leif Ericson Park reflects yet another of Brooklyn's sub-cultures—the sizable Scandinavian-American community that settled in Brooklyn from 1825 through the rest of that century. This park is dedicated to the Norse voyager who landed in northeastern North America nearly 500 years before Christopher Columbus.

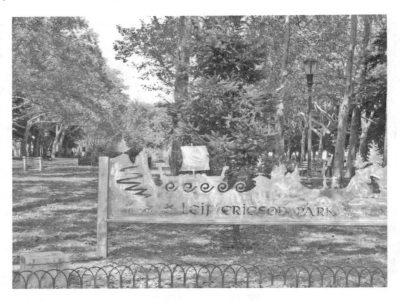

**Leif Ericson Park Entrance**

The park is decorated according to Norse themes. You might appreciate the water fountain at the entrance and restrooms further along at 5th Avenue. On-foot conditions are very pleasant, with plenty of shade and greenery.

At 7th Avenue, there is a somewhat complex dogleg diversion, in order to cross over Interstate 278. There are pedestrian lights so you do not have to compete with road traffic. On the other side of the highway, pick up 67th Street, and the continuation of Leif Ericson Park.

Keep following Leif Ericson Park on 67th Street until it ends at 3rd Avenue. Continue following 67th Street two short blocks to Owl's Head Park. There is a water fountain at the 67th Street entrance to this park. Negotiate this lovely park however you want—we found bearing left was easiest. You end up on the waterfront, with a view of Staten Island across the bay and, to the far right, the skyline of Manhattan and the Statue of Liberty.

Work your way to the southeast corner of the park at 68th Street. Here you find the start of a paved bike path. Follow that to 69th Street, and then turn right under the Shore Parkway to the American Veterans Memorial Pier.

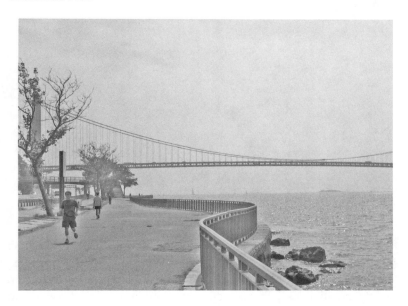

**The Brooklyn Shore Trail and Verrazano-Narrows Bridge**

Now you come to a wide, pleasant system of pedestrian and bicycle paths following the waterfront southward toward the Verrazano-Narrows Bridge. These paths can take you along the waterfront, under the bridge, and on as far as Bay Parkway, should you want to go that far. For this route we recommend leaving the shoreline before the bridge, and entering the local business and residential area, Bay Ridge. There is not a lot to see or do at Bay Parkway.

We suggest heading inland 1.3 miles after the pier at 92nd Street, where there is a convenient pedestrian bridge over the Shore Parkway. Follow 92nd Street to 3rd Avenue, one of Bay Ridge's two main streets. (4th Avenue is the other.) If you are ready for a break, 3rd Avenue has several good eating and drinking establishments, with the Verrazano-Narrows Bridge tower always in sight.

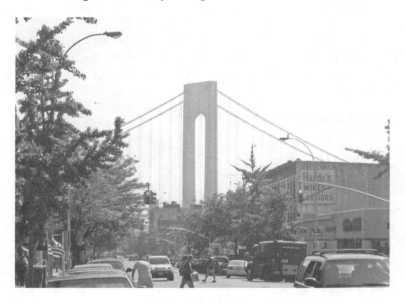

**3rd Avenue, Bay Ridge**

We liked Henry Grattan's at 3rd Avenue and 88th Street—an Irish Pub with medieval-style decoration and very good food. However, there are many other places to eat and drink around here—we have no doubt you will quickly find something to your liking. We dropped into a few places and enjoyed them all. An important point is that you will be among locals here—not tourists. Bay Ridge is an excellent place to feel the pulse of Brooklyn in the very pleasant atmosphere of local mid-market eating and drinking establishments.

To catch a subway home, go west to 4th Avenue at 86th or 95th Street. The trains from here will whiz you back to Downtown Brooklyn, or Manhattan, or … somewhere...

# Brooklyn to Coney Island

| Distance | 8.0 miles |
|---|---|
| Comfort | Good on-foot conditions. Expect other on-foot exercisers but no crowds. The route uses dedicated pedestrian or pedestrian/bicycle paths, plus sidewalks along a particularly pleasant, spacious parkway. OK for inline skating. |
| Attractions | Traverse Brooklyn's answer to Central Park, follow a wide runner-friendly parkway for 5.3 miles, experience suburban Brooklyn, and end at a famous amusement park and beach. |
| Convenience | Start at Grand Army Plaza in Brooklyn (or come here on foot from Lower Manhattan via the Brooklyn Bridge; add 3.5 miles). The No. 2 and 3 subway lines from Manhattan service Grand Army Plaza, and other lines have stops nearby. End at Coney Island. There are various subways from the Stillwell Avenue station at Coney Island back to Downtown Brooklyn or Manhattan. |
| Destination | The country's most famous amusement park and FUN area, Coney Island, including the historic Nathan's hot dog joint. There is plenty of fast food and the occasional better restaurant. |

Have you heard of Coney Island, but never quite got there? Here is your big opportunity, seeing more of Brooklyn and gaining some fitness on the way.

We present here a route from Grand Army Plaza to Coney Island. You can take the subway to Grand Army Plaza or, if you are happy to go the 11.5-mile distance, travel on-foot from Manhattan. With the latter option, follow the first part of our previous route to Grand Army Plaza.

Starting from Grand Army Plaza, negotiate lovely Prospect Park two miles to its southwest corner. (See our previous route for more details.) If you have been through here before, choose a different route through the park this time.

Exit the park at its southern rotary but this time, rather than taking Fort Hamilton Parkway, follow the signs to Ocean Parkway.

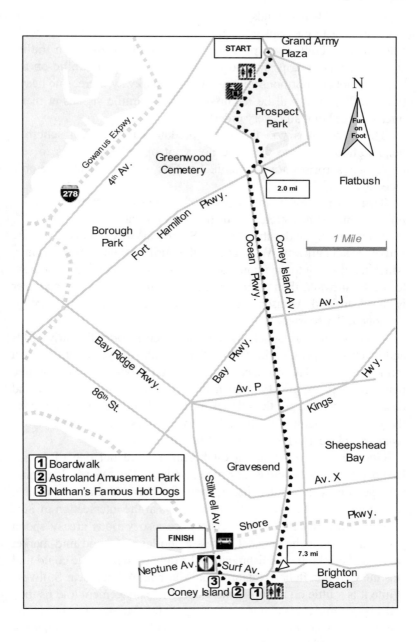

START

Grand Army Plaza

N

Fun on Foot

Prospect Park

Flatbush

2.0 mi

Gowanus Expwy.

278

4th Av.

Greenwood Cemetery

1 Mile

Fort Hamilton Pkwy.

Ocean Pkwy.

Coney Island Av.

Av. J

Borough Park

Bay Ridge Pkwy.

Bay Pkwy.

86th St.

Av. P

Kings

Hwy.

Sheepshead Bay

1 Boardwalk
2 Astroland Amusement Park
3 Nathan's Famous Hot Dogs

Gravesend

Av. X

Stillwell Av.

Pkwy.

Shore

FINISH

7.3 mi

Neptune Av.

Surf Av.

Brighton Beach

3 Coney Island 2 1

Ocean Parkway extends for 5.3 miles from here to the seashore. It is a particularly pleasant route for on-foot exercise. There are wide sidewalks on both edges plus additional pedestrian paths on traffic-separating nature strips for most of the way. There is traffic on the road, but not an enormous volume. Being a parkway, there is no heavy truck traffic. You will be required to wait at traffic signals at many intersections but it all is very orderly.

The route takes you through a predominantly Jewish suburban neighborhood. While there are not a lot of exciting things to see, unpleasant surprises are very unlikely. This is an excellent route on a nice day.

There is not much in the way of facilities, either restrooms or refreshments on this stretch, so be prepared for that.

After passing under the elevated Shore Parkway, you come to the end of Ocean Parkway. We suggest either turning right on Surf Avenue, which takes you into the main Coney Island area, or continuing straight to the Boardwalk, then turning right. The main sight you encounter is the Astroland Amusement park, complete with its 1927-vintage Cyclone roller coaster.

Coney Island was launched as an amusement resort in the early 1900s and reached its peak in the 1920s after the subway was built. Then, a million people a day would come here for fun. Today, it is nothing like that. The Depression, a 1944 fire at the Luna Park amusement park, and changing tastes and politics all took their toll. However, it is still fun for the young or young-at-heart, and operating rides such as the Cyclone make this place a living museum of fun activities.

Good eating and drinking establishments are not one of Coney Island's strengths. There is, of course, Nathan's Famous hot dog stand, still operating successfully since it opened in 1916. Nathan's is credited with originating the fast-food concept. It is at the intersection of Surf Avenue and Stillwell Avenue. There are also various greasy spoon joints throughout the area. There is a shortage of good mid-market eating and drinking establishments. The only such place we could find was the Carolina Italian restaurant on Mermaid Avenue near Stillwell. While it is a little on the up-market side, the management told us they had no qualms at all about welcoming untidy runners (which is the condition we were in at the time). So you will definitely not go hungry or thirsty around here. Alternatively, when you have seen enough, you can always catch the subway elsewhere, such as to Manhattan, where eating and drinking places abound.

The subway station is on Stillwell Avenue at the western end of the amusement park, one block inland from Surf Avenue.

If you like an eight-mile run, jog, or walk and also have nostalgia for old-style amusement parks, you will unquestionably find this route a winner!

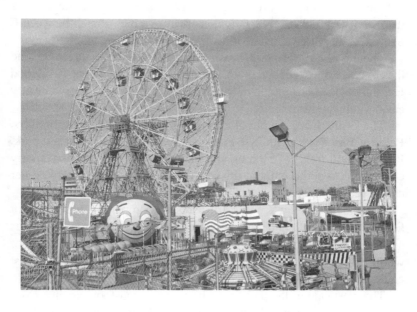

**Coney Island Amusement Park**

# Other Ideas

There are innumerable running routes in New York City. We have done our best to pick out those few routes that meet all our criteria well, including being convenient to central Manhattan.

Here are some other routes that we considered but did not quite make the cut. They might work fine for you, however.

There is a pedestrian and bicycle trail along the **East River** from E 63rd Street up to the Triboro Bridge at E 120th Street. It generally follows the heavily trafficked FDR Drive, apart from a nice stretch between E 81st and E 89th Streets, where it diverts to a level above the roadway.

There is also the **Hudson River** trail north of W 125th Street, beyond the coverage of our second route. This trail continues right up to Inwood Hill Park at the northern tip of Manhattan Island. You can conveniently catch a subway from there.

The Bronx has a couple of interesting parks for on-foot exercisers. **Pelham Bay Park**, with 2,764 acres, is New York City's largest park. It has several miles of running and hiking trails. It is not particularly convenient to get to without driving, although its southwestern corner can be reached by subway, at the end of the No. 6 Line.

**Van Cortlandt Park**, with 1,146 acres, is a comparatively convenient Bronx park to reach and has a number of attractions. Foremost, it has a very substantial area of wilderness with leafy forests and a lot of wildlife. We tried hard to construct a fun-on-foot route here but just could not satisfy all our criteria.

The west side of the park is the best part for on-foot exercise. You can get there easily by subway at the end of the No. 1 line. Then head north around the Parade Ground, past the Van Cortlandt House Museum (a historic site) and the Nature Center. At the Nature Center, you can pick up a trail map for the park. This map is essential if traversing the park for the first time, but it still does not make everything clear for the on-footer. In general, trails are not very well marked and several of the trails appearing on the map turn out to be of quite questionable quality.

However, if you stick to the west side of the park, you can have a nice four-to-five mile outing around a circuit extending into the Northwest Forest. After crossing Henry Hudson Parkway and entering the Northwest Forest area, we strongly recommend you follow the Cross Country Course, a trail marked with tortoise-and-hare signs for its length. Then, bearing eastward, you can pass Van Cordlandt Lake and the Van Cordlandt Golf Clubhouse (where you can stop for a snack and a drink). Then swing westward to get back to the subway station on Broadway.

The trail map includes the John Muir Nature Trail that takes you to the east side of the park to connect with other trails such as the Old Croton Aqueduct Trail, which can lead you back to the golf clubhouse. It can even take you further east to exits from the park on its east side. However, in our experience, we suggest you only attempt the John Muir Nature Trail if you have company and very limited expectations.

We have not covered **Staten Island**, which is not conveniently accessible on-foot from Manhattan or Brooklyn. Unfortunately, there is no pedestrian walkway on the Verrazano-Narrows Bridge. There is considerable interest in adding one and, if that were done, we would have some exciting options. For example, one could get to Staten Island via that bridge and return via the Staten Island Ferry. Maybe some day…

\* \* \* \*

For the day we spent in the Bronx's Van Cordlandt Park, Nola wore her Red Sox cap, despite this being the center of the New York Yankees world. This resulted in a few surprised looks, but more good-natured ribbing than anything else from the locals. New Yorkers are fun.

New York is unquestionably one of the most amazing cities in the world to visit. While most people know of the entertainment, fashions, historical sites, museums, local customs, and general hype of this city, not so many realize what a great place it is to get out and enjoy on-foot. This is absolutely not automobile land. Explore the Big Apple on foot and have fun!

# City of Brotherly Love

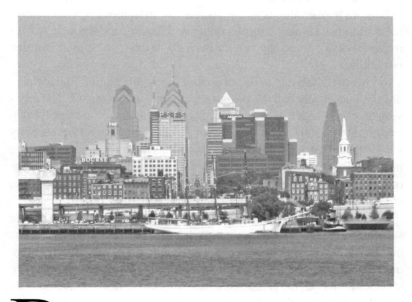

Birthplace of the United States, Philadelphia is packed with historic sites and memorabilia, including the room where the Declaration of Independence was issued in 1776 and the original U.S. Constitution was written in 1787. If Boston is where the Revolution started, Philadelphia is where it ended. In fact, there were more battles fought within a 50-mile radius of Philadelphia than in all of the New England colonies combined.

Philadelphia's appeal, however, goes far beyond its revolutionary period history. This city has much to offer visitors by way of museums, art venues, theater, and cultural and sporting events. It has many excellent restaurants and bars as well.

Located on the wide Delaware River, at the confluence with the attractive Schuylkill (pronounced *skoo-kil*) River, Philadelphia also has some very scenic on-foot terrain. Furthermore, Philadelphians rank high in on-foot enthusiasm. On the most popular recreational running or walking routes, you will encounter many health-conscious locals, weekdays and weekends alike. Having a mid-morning jog along Center City streets is also a normal activity. ("Center City" is Philly-speak for "downtown.")

Philadelphia weather is quite good for on-foot exercise. The average maximum temperature is in our desired 40-80 degrees Fahrenheit range for 8 months; January squeaks under at 39, and June through August make the 80's. There is precipitation 32% of days, so be ready for that possibility.

How safe is this city to be out on foot—possibly alone? Philadelphia has not historically had the best of reputations in this regard. The city's violent crime index is a quite high 13.8 (violent crimes per 1,000 inhabitants in 2003), compared with 5.8 for San Diego (the best city we visit) and 19.7 for Atlanta (the worst). However, conditions have improved in recent years, especially in Center City. If you venture out of Center City, you can encounter some questionable areas. Therefore, chart your course carefully and always use good street sense.

The public transit system is OK but nothing to be proud of. The subways are quite limited in their route coverage. For many purposes one needs to depend on the SEPTA Regional (R) trains, which are quite comprehensive in their routes, including an airport-to-downtown service. However, the R trains are more expensive than the average city transit system and their frequency is very poor—typically an hourly service on weekdays (off-peak), in some cases stretching to a 90-minute service on weekends. Be sure to pick up timetables and carry them with you.

I cannot express confidence in the reliability of the R trains. One train we were on came to a sudden stop when one of its overhead pantagraphs disintegrated, with an impressive fireworks display and many crashing noises. We consequently sat disabled for an hour and a half on the Schuylkill River rail bridge, until another train stopped to pick us up.

Everyone on board remained totally unphased through this entire incident, as if it happens every day. (Maybe it does.) The only sign of stress was in the young man on his cell phone trying to explain to his skeptical mom why he was neither at school nor at his after-school job. "Mom, you've got to believe me! I really have been stuck on the Schuylkill Bridge for the last hour!" I guess he had a few credibility issues at home...

\* \* \* \*

Now let us suggest a few specific on-foot routes that satisfy our usual criteria. We include a couple of short, central loops plus three longer runs out of the center.

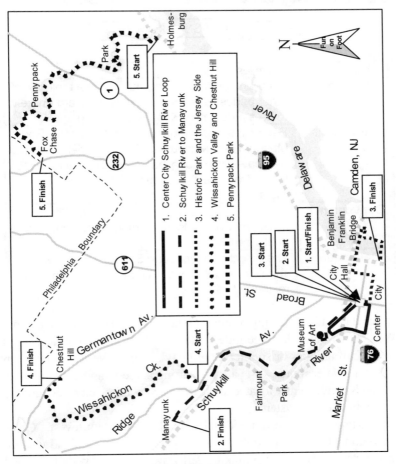

**Philadelphia Routes**

| Route | Distance |
|---|---|
| 1.  Center City Schuylkill River Loop | 3.3 miles |
| 2.  Schuylkill River to Manayunk | 7.9 miles |
| 3.  Historic Park and the Jersey Side | 4.1-to-5.6 miles |
| 4.  Wissahickon Valley and Chestnut Hill | 7.4 miles |
| 5.  Pennypack Park | 10.2 miles |

# Center City Schuylkill River Loop

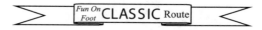

| Distance | 3.3 miles |
|---|---|
| **Comfort** | Excellent on-foot conditions.   Expect plenty of other pedestrians around but crowds are unlikely to be a problem.  OK for inline skating. |
| **Attractions** | Pass by several museums, including the Rodin Museum and Museum of Art.  Experience a nice new paved trail along the Schuylkill River in Center City.   Traverse the popular Rittenhouse Square District. |
| **Convenience** | A loop that starts and ends in Center City, close to downtown hotels, the Convention Center, and public transit. |
| **Destination** | The eclectic Rittenhouse Square District, with its variety of small shops, nice residences, and good restaurants and pubs. |

Let us start with something simple and short, but pleasant and interesting. We don't usually do three-mile routes, but this one is a great way to spend half an hour or so after a hard day's work. We'll also build on it in some later routes. It is a loop starting and ending near City Hall, which is conveniently located at the dead center of the city's geography and public transit system.

Starting at the western side of City Hall, head northwest.  Cross the road to JFK Plaza, go through that plaza, cross again, and you are at the start of Benjamin Franklin Parkway.  This is a wide tree-lined boulevard, with good pedestrian paths down both sides and the center as well. Follow this parkway to its end, negotiating Logan Circle on the way.

On this route, you pass by many of Philadelphia's prime art-world treasures. Here on Ben's Parkway, you even get to see some art treasures first hand. For example, if you use the right-hand sidewalk, you pass Rodin's *Thinker* outside the Rodin Museum.

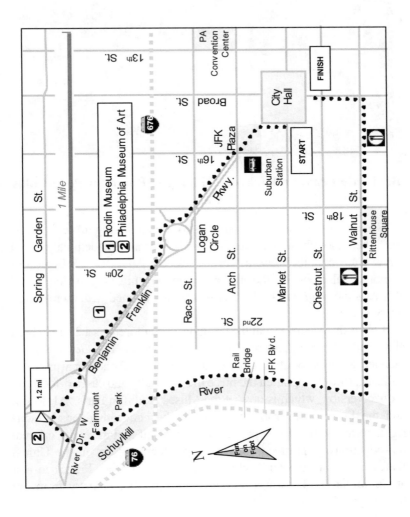

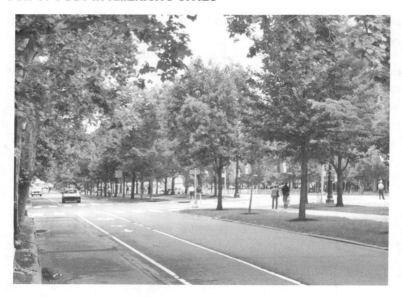

## Benjamin Franklin Parkway—Plenty of Room for People plus Cars

Seeing the *Thinker* inspired me to do some thinking myself. "How can it be," thought I, "that the *Thinker* is here in Philadelphia, when I know it furrows its brow in San Francisco's Palace of the Legion of Honor and also ponders the lawn at Columbia University in New York? Where is the *original Thinker*? Are we being conned with mere copies everywhere?"

I have since learned that the "original" sculpture was a 27-inch high clay model forming part of Rodin's larger design, *The Gates of Hell*, planned to sit above the doors of a museum in Paris that was never built. M. Rodin magnified the piece mechanically and cast a 6-feet high bronze version, which is now at the Museé Rodin in Paris. M. Rodin and the French Government, to whom he bequeathed posthumous rights to his work, also approved the casting of a number of "original reproductions." Thirteen "original reproductions" are in the United States, including the one right here and those in San Francisco and at Columbia U. I learnt a lot about the sculpting industry from my thinking on this run...

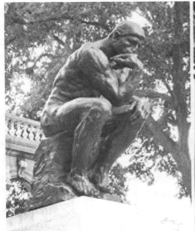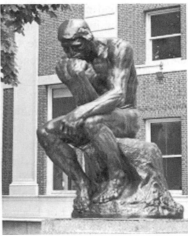

**Rodin's *Thinker* in Philadelphia and at Columbia U.**

The next major sight on the Benjamin Franklin Parkway is Philadelphia's famous Museum of Art. It houses over 300,000 pieces of art. However, to many, it is better known for its role in the Rocky movies.

Rocky, portrayed by Sylvester Stallone, concluded his pre-fight training here by running up the steps and celebrating triumphantly at the top. Getting back to sculpture, you might remember the Rocky statue at the top of those steps in later Rocky movies. The statue is real and stood above those steps for a while, donated by Stallone himself to the city. However, concerns about artistic taste and/or (my theory) a desire to hex the Philadelphia Flyers out of their post-1975 Stanley Cup drought, caused the powers-that-be to relocate it to the Spectrum in South Broad Street.

While you are here at the Museum of Art, you have the opportunity to join the tourists in repeating Rocky's run up the steps and posing for a celebratory photo at the top.

From the steps of the museum, head south towards the road overpass. Follow the street under the overpass. Cross River Dr. W to reach the bank of the Schuylkill River.

Take the paved trail towards the left, downstream. This trail traverses Schuylkill River Park, which is the beneficiary of recent rebuilding and re-landscaping, hence very pleasant. Continue under the rail bridge and the first two road bridges. At the next bridge, Chestnut Street, you have an opportunity to go up to the street level. The same is true at the following bridge, Walnut Street, and we suggest you climb the stairs there. There are plans to extend the trail further downstream to South Street. When that is complete, you will have an obvious way to extend this route by another mile.

Follow the sidewalk of Walnut Street back to the center of the city. You pass Rittenhouse Square on the way, and can divert through it if you wish. If you are interested in a food or beverage break, there are plenty of restaurants and pubs on Walnut Street. Our recommendation is to go to 15th Street then one block south to Locust Street. There you find Fado, one of the finest Irish pubs anywhere outside Ireland.

Where Walnut Street or Locust Street intersects Broad Street, turn left to get back to City Hall. If you feel like doing a few more miles, see our Historic Park and Jersey Side route, which you can tack straight onto this one.

# Schuylkill River to Manayunk

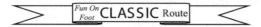

| Distance | 7.9 miles |
|---|---|
| Comfort | Excellent on-foot conditions. Expect plenty of pedestrians and cyclists around but crowds are unlikely to be a problem. OK for inline skating. |
| Attractions | Pass by several city sights, including the Rodin Museum, Museum of Art, Boathouse Row, Fairmount Water Works, and Lincoln statue. Most of the route is in a very pleasant riverside setting. |
| Convenience | Start in Center City, close to downtown hotels, the convention center, and public transit. Finish at the Manayunk R6 rail station, with comfortable transit back to the city (but service is not always very frequent so we recommend carrying an R6 timetable with you). |
| Destination | The town center of Manayunk, rich in antique stores and other small shops. There are several excellent wind-down restaurant/pubs. |

Philadelphia has an impressive urban park system comprising around 9,000 acres. Given the city's size, this compares favorably with New York City's 28,000 acres. The centerpiece of Philadelphia's parks system is Fairmount Park, an enormous outdoor asset. Fairmount Park, comprising over 8,700 acres, claims to be the largest urban park in the United States. It is over 10 times larger than New York's Central Park.

The main parts of Fairmount Park hug the Schuylkill River and Wissahickon Creek, a tributary of the Schuylkill. There are several excellent exercise routes through these areas.

For the first of our two routes based on Fairmount Park, we again assume a start at City Hall. Our recommended route is 7.9 miles, with an option to bail out at 5.7 miles. If you plan to take the train back from your excursion, we strongly recommend you drop into Suburban Station (near JFK Plaza and City Hall) before starting out, to pick up a timetable for the R6 train (get the R7 and R8 timetables too while there—you might need them for later routes).

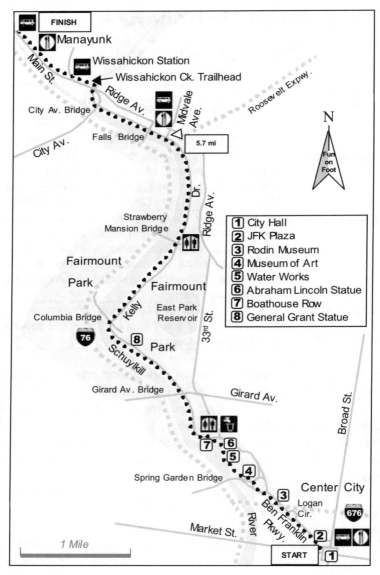

Follow the course of our first route to the Museum of Art. Keep to the left-hand side of the Museum of Art and follow the street under the traffic overpass to the Schuylkill River. Then head to the right, upstream. (Note the variation from our first route where we headed to the left, downstream.) While you can go up the river on the western bank, the eastern bank is the more pleasant, being away from the Interstate highway. Therefore, we recommend that you not cross the river here.

You soon come to the Fairmount Water Works, yet another significant piece of Philadelphian history. The Water Works went into operation in 1815 as a system to deliver water citywide for purposes of drinking, sanitation, and fire fighting. According to the city's information sources, Philadelphia led most U.S. cities in the provision of such services by a matter of decades. Furthermore, Philadelphia provided such services in style, complete with an installation characterized by its neoclassical architecture. The Water Works served the city until 1909 when its technology became obsolete, but it has since been preserved in various guises, including that of an aquarium in the first half of the 20th century.

From the Water Works, you also get an excellent view of one of Philadelphia's most picturesque architectural sights—Boathouse Row. The ten rowing clubs based in these Victorian style boathouses comprise the Schuylkill Navy, which was founded in 1858 and is considered the nation's oldest amateur athletic association. In 1887 the Athletic Club of the Schuylkill Navy started the Amateur Athletic Union of the United States. The rowing clubs based here are as active today as ever, and host several major regattas in spring and summer.

Philadelphia's surprises in the history department (and the sculpture department) just never cease to amaze. After passing the Water Works and continuing on the trail upstream towards Boathouse Row, one suddenly bumps into a statue of Abraham Lincoln, located somewhat aimlessly and irreverently by the side of the road. It so happens that this statue is the oldest known statue of Lincoln, created in 1871, six years after his assassination.

The trail from this point on follows Kelly Drive, the main road route up the Schuylkill on its east bank. This road is dedicated to one of Philadelphia's prominent families, which includes Grace Kelly (the late Princess of Monaco) as a member. Just under a mile from the Museum of Art, after the Lloyd Hall recreational facility, you arrive at Boathouse Row. The trail skirts the backs of the boathouses. There are public restrooms and a basic café here.

For the next 3.6 miles up the Schuylkill, we suggest you simply relax and enjoy the lovely on-foot conditions. The scenery is very pleasant, and you can expect the company of many other pedestrians and cyclists. There is a paved bike path all the way and, in some parts, a separate gravel running trail or an unpaved edge adopted by the on-foot community.

Along this stretch, you pass the Girard Avenue, Columbia, and Strawberry Mansion bridges. There are helpful signs along the way that help you track your mileage progress, and also point you to some of the preserved mansions that Fairmount Park hosts. You also pass yet another famous and impressive statue—of General Ulysses Grant—at Fountain Green Drive.

At 3.6 miles from Boathouse Row you come to Midvale Avenue, where you can cross Kelly Drive at a traffic light. You might choose to take a break or even bail out of the excursion here, if you need to, although we strongly encourage you to keep going another two miles. A short distance up Midvale there are various acceptable food and drink joints such as Johnny Manana's Mexican grill. The East Parks R6 Station is also right here so, subject to the R train schedule, you can easily get back to Center City.

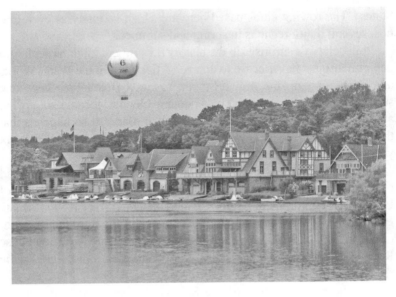

**Boathouse Row**

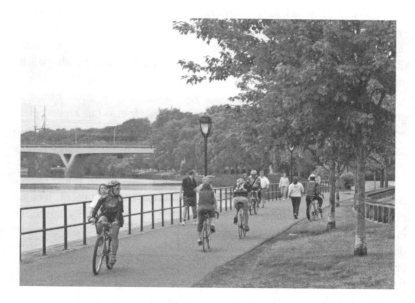

### The Schuylkill Trail—You Will Not be Lonely Here

If you're still with us, follow the river trail a little further to where Wissahickon Creek meets the river and where Kelly Drive ends. Keep bearing to the left and follow the creek around until you hit the road bridge over the creek—the road is Ridge Avenue. Cross the creek on this bridge.

There is an important trail junction here. If you crossed Ridge Avenue, you would find the trailhead of the Wissahickon Valley Trail System. Alternatively, you can continue up the Schuylkill along Ridge Avenue. For the route we are presently describing, we shall assume the latter alternative. However, a later route features the Wissahickon, so you may want to note this as a point to return to another day.

For now, we propose continuing up the Schuylkill a little way to a very interesting town that we think you will appreciate.

Less than a quarter mile along Ridge Avenue you can see on the cliff bluffs on the northern side of the road an ivy-covered, almost medieval-castle-like, entrance to a train station. This is the Wissahickon station on the R6 line. You do not want to use this now, but take note, since it may prove useful in getting you to or from the Wissahickon trailhead some other day.

Follow the road a little further and you come to a left exit with a sign welcoming you to "Main Street Manayunk." Follow this exit. The next half-mile or so takes you through the outskirts of Manayunk—quite dull and uninspiring. However, as the town starts to take shape, the situation improves big time.

Manayunk is an attractive, touristy town, with a good range of antique stores and other browsing destinations. It also has an excellent collection of pubs and restaurants. You might, by now, be ready to hunker down for a good brunch, lunch, or just a well-earned beverage break.

The first place you encounter on the way in, and a good choice too, is the Manayunk Brewing Company. This establishment, located on the old canal towpath just after Shurs Lane, has a very attractive environment, especially the outdoor canal-side patio on a summer day. It also has an excellent food and beverage menu and regular entertainment. Continuing further into town, you come to many other fine establishments. We had a nice lunch at Zesty's, a Greek cuisine bar/ restaurant. Other places, including Bourbon Blue, Thomas' Restaurant, Le Bus Manayunk, and the Bayou Bar and Grill all seemed very good too, and we would not discourage you from trying those.

When done with your eating, drinking, and shopping, take the R6 train back to Center City. The Manayunk Station is at Main and Carson Streets, convenient to all the central establishments. Remember the issue with the frequency of R trains, though, and judiciously use the timetable you picked up prior to heading for the station.

# Historic Park and the Jersey Side

| Distance | 4.1-to-5.6 miles |
|---|---|
| Comfort | Use street sidewalks for the first 1.5 miles in Center City; expect many other pedestrians around for that part. After that, use the bridge walkway/bikeway and dedicated pedestrian paths on the Jersey side. Pedestrians might be sparse on the second half of the route at off-peak times but you could encounter crowds if you hit a special event. OK for inline skating if you don't mind the substantial uphill and downhill of the bridge. |
| Attractions | Pass by the city's most historic sites, including Independence Hall, the Liberty Bell pavilion, Christ Church Burial Ground, and the Philadelphia Mint. See impressive views of the Delaware River and surrounds while crossing the Benjamin Franklin suspension bridge. See the classic view of Center City from the Jersey side. Pass the New Jersey Aquarium and visit it if you wish. Have a pleasant and scenic ferry ride back to Penn's Landing. |
| Convenience | A loop that starts and ends in Center City, handy to downtown hotels, the Convention Center, and public transit. Note, however, that it involves a ferry trip, so takes longer than the distance suggests. Also, to complete the loop back to the City Hall or Convention Center, add roughly 1.5 miles, giving 5.6 miles total. If desired, you can tack this route onto our first route (add 3.3 miles). |
| Destination | Historic Penn's Landing, with a choice of great restaurants and pubs nearby for winding down. You can also go on to visit the Historic Park tourist destinations. |

Let us now describe a short route that is interesting and a little different. The route we describe is 4.1 miles, but that ends at Penn's Landing. Add 1.5 miles to complete the loop back to the start.

This route was developed with attractions foremost in mind. The idea is to string together five main elements:

(1) Famous Independence National Historic Park;
(2) The impressive Benjamin Franklin suspension bridge across the Delaware;
(3) The riverside trail in New Jersey, which offers an excellent panorama of the Center City skyline;
(4) A feet-up ferry ride back across the Delaware; and
(5) (Optional) A wrap-up meal, drinks, and chat with the locals at a friendly Center City Irish pub.

This route may take longer than you would think, because of the ferry wait (not to mention the pub stop). It is not the sort of route for training to run a marathon, but it sure makes for a very pleasant afternoon out.

We again assume a start at City Hall. There are various ways to get to the Benjamin Franklin Bridge approach. The following 1.6-mile route from City Hall is one. First you need to get across town to 5th Street. We suggest using Walnut Street, which is fairly wide and lightly trafficked. From City Hall, go three blocks south to Walnut then take Walnut roughly eight blocks east. On the way, note No. 1116 Walnut—Moriarty's Pub—one of the best Irish pubs around; you might like to return here later.

When you reach Washington Square West, for a pleasant little diversion, take the southeast-heading path into Washington Square, passing the Tomb of the Unknown Soldier. At the center of the square, turn left taking the northeast-heading path back to Walnut at 6th Street. Cross both streets at this intersection and you are at the southwest corner of Independence Square. Continue to 5th Street also known as Independence Mall East. Turn left heading north.

5th Street takes you past the top historic sites of this city. At Chestnut Street you pass Old City Hall and, next to it, Independence Hall, where the Declaration of Independence and U.S. Constitution originated. Beyond Independence Hall is Congress Hall, home to the House of Representatives and Senate from 1790 to 1800 and where the Bill of Rights was ratified in 1791. Then you pass the Liberty Bell pavilion; Christ Church Burial Ground where Benjamin Franklin rests; and the Philadelphia U.S. Mint, the world's largest mint, which has been in operation since the inception of the republic.

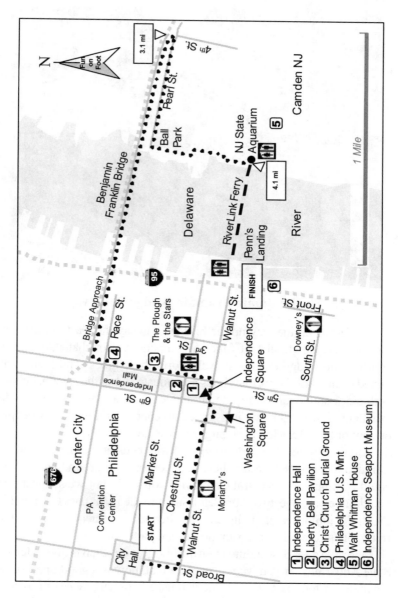

After passing the Mint, cross Race Street and keep going straight ahead. You come to the entrance to the southern walkway/bikeway of the Benjamin Franklin Bridge.

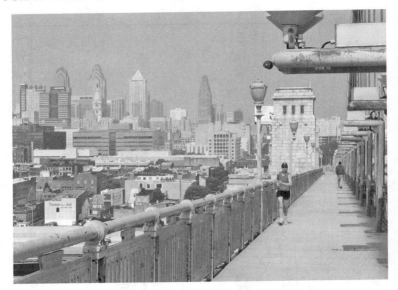

## The Benjamin Franklin Bridge Walkway

The grade on the way up the bridge is, to say the least, noticeable, but the easy downhill that follows compensates for that. All in all, crossing the bridge on foot is well worth the effort. The scenery is mixed—much of the surroundings are industrial, but the river itself and both sides southward are quite attractive. You are also treated to an excellent view of Center City. Expect to encounter a few other people on foot or bicycle. However, large crowds are unlikely.

After 1.5 miles, the pedestrian walkway ends at North 4$^{th}$ Street in Camden, New Jersey. Stairs here take you back to ground level. You could continue on to central Camden if you wish, but we suggest that you double back westward on Pearl Street to the river, pass Campbell's Field, the junior league ballpark, and then turn left heading down the river. There is a wide, pleasant pedestrian path here.

One mile after descending from the bridge, you reach the New Jersey State Aquarium. If you want to explore that, now is a good time, since the main on-foot part of this route is finished. Other places of possible interest around here are the Wiggins Waterfront Park and Amphitheater, Walt Whitman House (three blocks up Mickle Boulevard from the amphitheater), and the Blockbuster-Sony Entertainment Center.

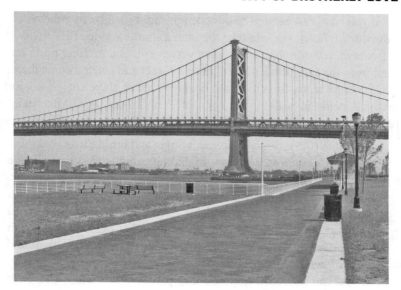

**The Spacious Jersey-side Pedestrian Path**

Adjacent to the aquarium is the RiverLink Ferry that can take you back to Pennsylvania. When we were last there, the ferry ran on a 40-minute schedule and was a bit expensive—$6 for a return ticket, with no one-way fare offered. However, it is very pleasant and you get to see the sights on both sides of the Delaware during the crossing.

The ferry takes you to Penn's Landing. William Penn, an English Quaker, was granted a parcel of land here in 1682, as payment for a debt the English Crown owed his father. Penn established a settlement and named it Philadelphia, derived from the Greek for *brotherly love*. Philadelphia grew rapidly, becoming the second largest English-speaking city in the world just before the American Revolution. Penn's Landing is where Penn first came ashore.

Having retraced Penn's steps and alighted at Penn's Landing, you have the opportunity to explore the nation's maritime history at the Independence Seaport Museum.

To get straight back to the City Hall and Convention Center vicinity on foot, work your way through Penn's Landing in a due westerly direction and you come to a pedestrian overpass over Interstate 95, taking you to Walnut Street. Follow Walnut Street roughly 1.5 miles.

If you have had enough on-foot action and want a cushy ride back to a downtown hotel, you can take the tourist shuttle service PHLASH. It is frequent, comfortable, and costs a very nominal fare. Bear north and west from the ferry dock up to Chestnut Street and catch the bus there.

If you are ready for a food and beverage break, there are some good establishments in walking distance of Penn's Landing. After much research, we can recommend three fine Irish pubs near here:

- *Downey's* (0.5 mile away at South Street and Front Street) has great food and an impressive décor, including genuine wood paneling, a bar imported from Ireland, and a zillion antiques and memorabilia. Sunday brunch is offered. From the ferry dock, head south past the cruiser *USS Olympia* and the submarine *USS Becuna*—you can tour these if you wish. Keep going until you see a pedestrian bridge over Interstate 95. Take this bridge to Downey's. West and north of here, there is a lively area for entertainment and shopping, so you can move on to interesting places afterwards. The walk back to City Hall or the Convention Center from Downey's is about two miles. You can plot a course through Historic Society Hill, with its federal period town houses.

- *The Plough and the Stars* (0.4 mile away in 3rd Street near Chestnut Street) is located in the historically preserved Corn Exchange Building, dated back to the early 20th century. The food, drink, and company are great. Saturday and Sunday brunch are served. Bear north and west from the ferry dock up to Chestnut Street. Take Chestnut Street to 3rd Street and turn right to The Plough and the Stars. This pub has the advantage of being close to Independence National Historic Park so you can easily go on to explore these sights later if you wish.

- *Moriarty's* (1.0 mile away at 1116 Walnut Street) has charm, a warm inviting ambiance, a comprehensive food menu, and 30 draft beers. Follow our on-foot directions back to the City Hall and Convention Center vicinity via Walnut Street.

We expect you will have fun on this route. But it is time to move on to something a bit more strenuous.

# Wissahickon Valley and Chestnut Hill

| Distance | 7.4 miles |
|---|---|
| Comfort | Good running/jogging conditions, except for some hiking trail conditions near the start and end. Generally plenty of pedestrians around, but no crowds. Expect some parts of the trail to be devoid of other pedestrians. Not suitable for inline skating. |
| Attractions | An escape from city life, mainly in a wilderness setting, far away from cars. It is mostly shady, following a creek through a nature reserve. Signs along the route highlight several points of historic interest. There is a very pleasant and attractive township at the end. |
| Convenience | Start and finish at SEPTA rail stations, with comfortable transit from and to Center City. Start by taking the R6 train to Wissahickon Station, roughly six miles northwest of City Hall. Finish at Chestnut Hill on the R8 line. (We recommend carrying an R8 timetable with you.) |
| Destination | The lovely township of Chestnut Hill, with good pub/restaurants such as the Chestnut Grill and Solaris Grill. There are many antique stores and other small shops. |

The Wissahickon Valley is a very popular area with Philadelphia locals for running, jogging, walking, cycling, or generally escaping from the pressures of city life. Most locals would approach a Wissahickon on-foot excursion by driving to and parking at an access point, doing a suitable out-and-back loop, and then driving home. That is a fine approach. However, if you want to detach from the auto and follow our usual formula, here is what we suggest.

Start from the Wissahickon trailhead on Ridge Avenue at Wissahickon Creek. You can get to it by taking the R6 train to Wissahickon Station then trekking southeastward down the road about a quarter of a mile. Alternatively, travel here on foot (roughly six miles) following our Schuylkill River route description. The route we describe here covers 7.4 miles in all, ending in the lovely town of Chestnut Hill, where you can obtain rest and sustenance and catch an R train back to Center City.

## FUN OF FOOT IN AMERICA'S CITIES

This route has the occasional stretch that you might consider hiking conditions, but most of it is suitable for running and jogging.

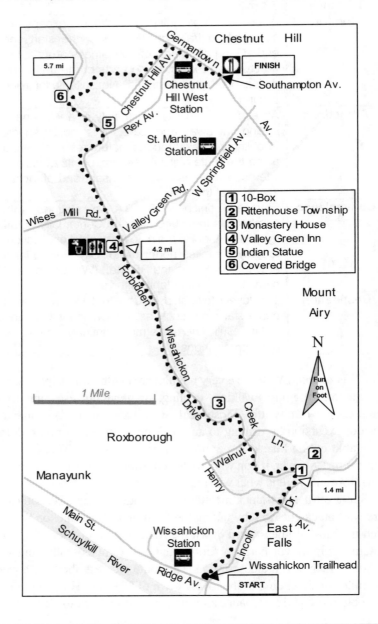

The first 1.4 miles follow the creek on its northern side up to 10-Box, which is the southernmost end of Forbidden Drive. This path, while environmentally pleasant and adequately removed from the automobile traffic on Lincoln Drive across the creek, is not particularly good underfoot. Think of this part more as a hiking trail, although you can certainly run parts of it.

10-Box is a relic from the 1940s. It was originally a guard station house, which subsequently became #10 of a set of ten phone boxes on the Wissahickon. On reaching 10-Box, our recommended route follows Forbidden Drive northward.

---

**VARIATION**

If you keep following Lincoln Drive and the small creek for another quarter mile, you come to Rittenhouse Township. William Rittenhouse was the first Mennonite minister in America. In 1690, shortly after William Penn's landing, Rittenhouse's colonial community built their first paper mill right here. The next generation added to the mill and by the 1850s there were forty buildings in the town. Seven remain today. Scientist David Rittenhouse was born here in 1732. Guided tours are available on weekends.

---

Forbidden Drive is a gravel path following Wissahickon Creek for about five miles through beautiful overhanging trees, with little waterfalls running down the face of rocks along the way. Forbidden Drive was originally a road, completed in 1856. It became a turnpike in 1869. The very exciting thing is that, thanks to the evolution of the area's road system plus a sense of environmental responsibility, the road was closed to all traffic in 1899. Hence the name: Forbidden Drive. It was debated for another 30 years whether to make it a new road route—an expressway, in fact. This debate spawned the 1924 formation of the Friends of the Wissahickon, an association that today still nurtures the Wissahickon Valley's environment while fostering people presence. The non-automobile people won the day and driving is still forbidden. The walkers, runners, and cyclists of Philadelphia are thereby blessed with an outstanding, relaxing, recreational asset.

Forbidden Drive has plenty of trail width to accommodate everyone. It also has various signposts along the way, pointing out interesting historical and environmental features.

---

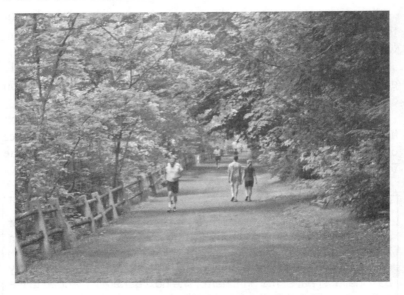

### Forbidden Drive—Philadelphians' Great Escape

From 10-Box, head up Forbidden Drive 2.8 miles to the Valley Green Inn. We would caution against exiting the park on-foot to the east earlier than the Valley Green Inn, since the suburbs in those parts are a bit questionable.

The Valley Green Inn, built in 1850, is a charming restaurant, with colonial era décor, sponsored by the Friends of the Wissahickon. There are restrooms and water here. Table service lunch and dinner are served at the restaurant, but you cannot really drop in for a snack or drink.

You can exit the park on-foot at Valley Green Road if you need to, but the route is not pedestrian-friendly. You need to skirt roads without sidewalks, albeit with light vehicle traffic. If you must exit here, follow Valley Green Road then West Springfield Avenue to St. Martins R8 line station. There are no food or drink outlets this way.

We recommend you continue northbound on Forbidden Drive a little further.

One mile from the Valley Green Inn you come to a major path off to the right—Rex Avenue—and yet another impressive piece of Philadelphian sculpture, in the form of an Indian statue perched high above the trail. The statue, portraying a Lenape warrior, was carved in 1902.

You can exit up Rex Avenue to Chestnut Hill if you wish, but, having come this far, we suggest you continue a little further to the covered bridge. This is the last of five such covered bridges originally in the Wissahickon Valley and the only one still standing. It is in excellent shape, thanks to a 1999 restoration.

You can continue on Forbidden Drive a further mile if you wish, but we recommend crossing the covered bridge and heading for Chestnut Hill at this point. Going further north is not very helpful if you ultimately want to get to Chestnut Hill on foot, since you will be forced onto some quite pedestrian-unfriendly roads. In particular, avoid Bells Mill Road, which has no sidewalk and quite heavy traffic.

After crossing the covered bridge, follow the main trail up, ignoring the various side trails on the way. The trail is sometimes a little steep and not the best underfoot so, if you have been running or jogging, you might want to treat this as a cool-down hike.

The trail ends at Chestnut Hill Avenue. Turn left and follow this street along a good sidewalk to Germantown Avenue. Turn right, walk a block, and enter one of the most gorgeous town centers you will find anywhere.

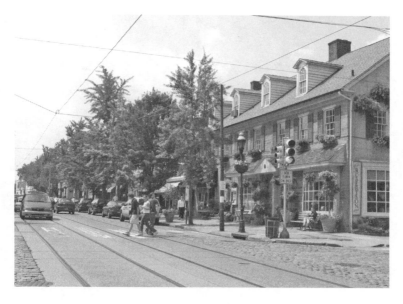

**Chestnut Hill—As Lovely as Towns Get**

Watch for the Chestnut Hill West train station on the right after Rex Avenue. Remember it if you want to take a train back to Philadelphia. However, if you feel like a food or beverage break or want to see more of the town, keep going east on Germantown Avenue.

The good eating and drinking happens a few blocks further along, at the intersection with Southampton Avenue. There are two good establishments here. We loved the Chestnut Grill, an independent restaurant/bar in the Chestnut Hill Hotel building. It has a very pleasant bar, plus outdoor dining along the hotel's front patio. The Solaris Grill, virtually across the street, is another excellent establishment and offers a Sunday brunch.

After enjoying the fare of either of these establishments, check out the timetable for the R8 train and plan your departure time from the restaurant accordingly. The last thing you want to do right now is waste an hour waiting on the platform. The Chestnut Hill West station is back along Germantown Avenue near Rex Avenue.

# Pennypack Park

| Distance | 10.2 miles |
|---|---|
| Comfort | Good running/jogging conditions on a paved bicycle/pedestrian trail, except for some street sidewalks near the start and end. Expect some other pedestrians around, but no crowds. Some parts of the trail may be devoid of other pedestrians. There is little water on the way so carry your own. Generally OK for inline skating. |
| Attractions | An escape from the crowds and traffic of the city, mainly in a wilderness setting. It is attractive and shady, following a creek through a nature reserve. There is considerable wildlife and no cars to bother you. |
| Convenience | Start and finish at SEPTA rail stations, with comfortable transit from and to Center City. Start by taking the R7 train to Holmesburg Junction, roughly seven miles northeast of City Hall. Finish at Fox Chase, the terminus of the R8 line. |
| Destination | The town of Fox Chase and the Blue Ox Brauhaus, an amazingly authentic Bavarian restaurant/bar. |

Our final route takes you far away from the city's crowds and traffic, into wooded terrain with plenty of wildlife, but with a well-groomed, paved trail its entire length. Its only detraction is in the convenience factor since, like the Wissahickon route, it depends on R trains to get there and back.

Take the R7 Trenton train to Holmesburg Junction. I must warn you that the scenery on the train trip is probably the worst found on the continent. Don't let that get you down, though—just use the trip as an opportunity for reading this book.

After alighting at the station, take Rhawn Street a block to the left to Torresdale Avenue. This is not the prettiest area in the world but you will soon be through it. Take Torresdale to the right. Pass trailheads on both sides of the road just before the bridge over Pennypack Creek. Continue across the bridge and take the paved trail to the left after the bridge. This is the main trail northward, paved for its full 8.4-mile length. Expect to pass a reasonable number of pedestrians and cyclists, and the occasional picnicking family. The trail is mostly shady, with considerable wildlife around.

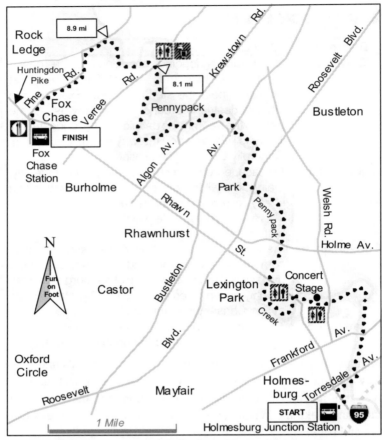

At Frankford Avenue, 0.4 mile from Torresdale, you have to cross the street. There is a pedestrian crossing a short distance to the right to help with that. After that, there are no more street crossings for the entire route, just underpasses—savor that aspect of this route!

After the Welsh Road underpass, you come to a concert stage, a venue for regular summer concerts. After that, cross the creek via a footbridge and you come to a trail fork.

Both paths ultimately lead you to the same place. Take the left path to follow the creek or the right path for a slightly shorter route but with some grades. The latter option also takes you near restrooms. When the trail emerges and starts following a street, you will come to a traffic signal and pedestrian crossing. If you cross here, you will find restrooms at the rear of the parking lot.

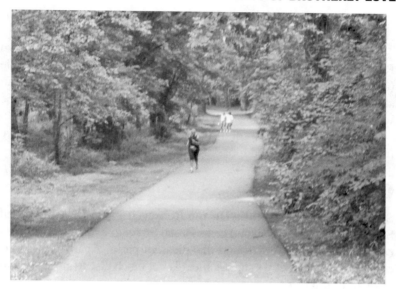

## Peace and Quiet in Pennypack Park

Continue on the trail to Verree Road. The park maps show an environmental center here, but we found it difficult to get to and closed on the summer Sunday we were there. Forget that one.

After crossing Verree, you encounter restrooms and a water fountain next to the trail.

Continue to Pine Road. Exit the park here and follow the left hand sidewalk of Pine Road 1.3 miles to the Huntingdon Pike. Here you are close to the Fox Chase R train station.

However, after that long run, jog, or walk, you are maybe more interested in visiting one of the country's most amazing eating and drinking establishments. Pine Road leads you straight to the Blue Ox Brauhaus. This is a Bavarian restaurant and bar, more authentic than you could imagine. The proprietor is native from Munich, so he really knows how to run such an establishment. The décor is Bavarian, the food is Bavarian, the beer is Bavarian, the music is Bavarian, and many of the staff are Bavarian. There is brunch on Saturday and Sunday with offerings such as a Bavarian breakfast, crepes, potato pancakes, and, of course, a bratwurst and sauerkraut sandwich. This is an amazing place and we highly recommend it.

There are some other pub and restaurant choices around here as well.

The Fox Chase R8 station is a couple of hundred yards away, down Rhawn Street. Before leaving the restaurant, check your R8 timetable (or ask the restaurant staff for the times). The R8 service frequency can stretch to 90 minutes on weekends so don't head for the station at the wrong time.

This route consumes a solid half-day, but is well worth it if you have the time and feel the need for escape from city life.

# Other Ideas

South of the city is **Franklin Delano Roosevelt Park**. Take the Broad Street subway to Pattison and cross Broad Street to enter the Park. You can do a 1.6-mile loop around this pleasant park. Apart from sports complexes (and Rocky's statue), there is not much else to attract you to this part of town.

Another park in the Fairmount Park system is **Cobbs Creek Park**, west of Center City. You can get there via the Market Street subway. There are some on-foot trails, but it is not as well developed as other parts of the Fairmount Park system  However, there are plans under way to extend the trail system in the near future, so this may become an interesting option.

If you are prepared to venture further out of Philadelphia, consider **Valley Forge National Historic Park**. This park, of over 3,600 acres, is where, in the winter of 1778, Washington and his troops survived through some of the worst winter conditions experienced in the Revolution. The park is reachable on foot from Center City via the Valley Forge Bike Trail, which continues up the Schuylkill River from where we were in Manayunk. However, Valley Forge is over 20 miles from Center City, so somewhat beyond the model for our usual routes.

* * * *

There is no doubt that Philadelphia is an excellent destination for spending time out on foot, gaining fitness, soaking up history and culture, and enjoying yourself at the same time. However, it is now time for us to move on...

Have phun in Philly!

# 5

# National Capital

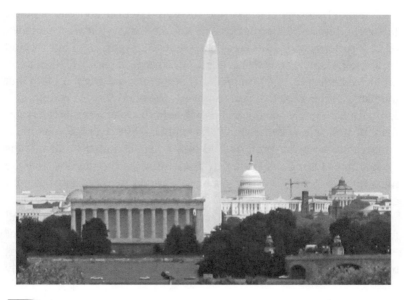

R unning is an important fundamental part of life in the nation's capital, Washington DC, and I don't just mean running for office and running for cover. The fitness kind of running is also prominent, thanks to the emphasis and exemplary healthy lifestyles demonstrated by many of our Presidents. Notable among these are Jimmy Carter who averaged 6 miles a day, the first George Bush who led the press corps on daily three-mile runs, Bill Clinton who was an eight-minute miler and snarled up the traffic regularly with his on-road runs, and the fastest president of all to date, George W. Bush, who ran the 1993 Houston Marathon in 3:44—a very classy performance indeed![1]

1　　　　Source: Lee Michaelides, *Runner's World*, October 2002.

This type of attitude at the top naturally works its way right down the inside-the-Beltway tree, with the consequence that Washingtonians are great on-foot enthusiasts. Add to that the tourist factor. Washington, with its outstanding set of tourist attractions, draws enormous numbers of visitors. Since many of the attractions are relatively close to each other, a good number of the tourists even realize they have a great opportunity to sightsee on foot, especially in the federal triangle and National Mall precincts. All in all, Washington is a city of enormous outdoor on-foot action.

Let us check out some of the inherent comfort and convenience factors in this city. In terms of safety, the city has a violent crime index of 15.7 (offenses per 1,000 residents in 2003)—quite high but it could be worse (Atlanta is our worst, at 19.7). There are parts of DC, mainly on the eastern side, that you probably want to avoid when on foot, but they are not the attractive parts anyway. Weather-wise, Washington is fairly friendly to the on-foot enthusiast—similar to or a smidgeon better than Boston, New York, and Philadelphia. The average maximum temperature is in our preferred 40-to-80 degrees range in all months except June through August. In those summer months the average maximum is in the 80's, suggesting you might want to start out a bit earlier in the day.

Given these environmental conditions, the tourist attractions, and the city's location on the attractive Potomac River (and with a major embedded park, Rock Creek Park), one gets strong up-front indications that some great on-foot experiences lie in wait here. That is absolutely true!

Washington's road traffic system is generally a nightmare. There is nothing particularly special about the street geography or the driving style but there always seems to be citywide gridlock. In contrast, the city's subway system—the Metro—is truly a national treasure. It is modern and clean, with broad region-wide coverage; and even the ticketing system is well designed and works! This is one of the advantages of a subway system constructed from scratch only about 30 years ago, compared with the dinosaurs in certain other major U.S. cities.

There are a couple of minor cautions for on-foot exercisers in DC. First, be careful not to get overly entangled with the sightseeing destinations, unless you can get out early morning before the sightseers emerge. One of your biggest hazards can be the sightseers who tend to move very slowly and often flock together in large numbers.

Another point to note: Washington is surprisingly deficient in the availability of water fountains along its pedestrian and cycling trails, so it pays to give a little extra attention to carrying adequate water on a longer route on a warm day.

To best satisfy our comfort/attractions/convenience/ destination formula, we decided to include some routes close to the central tourist action but also a couple of routes that take you out of the tourist chaos and offer you comparative peace, quiet, and escape. The latter routes have their fair share of other runners, joggers, and walkers, but those folk are, by and large, Washington locals rather than tourists. It will also become quickly obvious how you can mix elements of these various routes to create your own.

| Route | Distance |
|---|---|
| 1. National Mall and the Potomac | 4.9 miles |
| 2. Potomac Parks and Arlington | 8.0 miles |
| 3. Mount Vernon Trail to Alexandria | 10.0 miles |
| 4. Rock Creek Park to Georgetown | 6.0 miles |

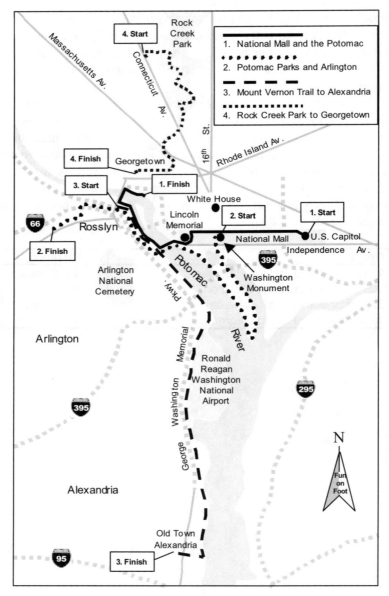

**Washington Routes**

# National Mall and the Potomac

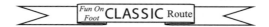

| Distance | 4.9 miles |
|---|---|
| Comfort | Excellent underfoot conditions and plenty of other on-foot exercisers around you. There may be some crowds on the first half, but generally there is enough space to bypass them. Not suitable for inline skating. |
| Attractions | Pass the Washington Monument, National WWII Memorial, Vietnam Veterans Memorial, Lincoln Memorial and other national attractions. Then escape the crowds for some exercise along the Potomac, see the C&O Canal, and end at a lively riverside eating and drinking spot. |
| Convenience | Start near the U.S. Capitol, within easy walking distance of hotels in the Federal Triangle or L'Enfant Plaza vicinities, or take the Metro to Federal Center SW (Blue and Orange Lines) or L'Enfant Plaza (Green and Yellow Lines). End at Georgetown or Washington Harbor within easy walking distance of Foggy Bottom and Dupont Circle, or take a Metro (Blue and Orange Lines) elsewhere. |
| Destination | Choose between Georgetown, with its historic sights, restaurants, and shops, and Washington Harbour, with several good restaurant/bars with outdoor patios on the Potomac riverfront. Tourist sights in the West Mall area are also convenient to here. |

The National Mall, which knits together many of the capital's most revered monuments, is one of the most famous urban green-spaces in the world. Because of its huge width, it is even runnable, despite the massive numbers of tourists who flock here. Therefore, we had no choice but to base our first route on the National Mall. Better still, it turns out we can tack on a couple of other ideas that make for an excellent quality overall on-foot exercise experience. The route described here is a modest 4.9 miles—not very stressing but a great way to fill in an hour or two at the end of a day in which indoor activities or travel have consumed your time.

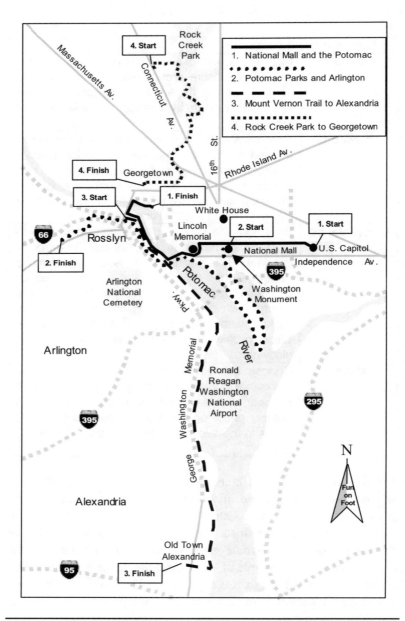

---

**VARIATION**

If you are staying in a hotel in the Georgetown, Foggy Bottom, Dupont Circle, McPherson Square, or Federal Triangle vicinities, you can easily turn this into a circle route from your hotel by tacking on the street-sidewalk segments to the start and back from the finish. This will add roughly two miles, giving a seven-mile route overall.

---

Start in front of the U.S. Capitol, which can be easily reached from downtown Washington on-foot or from Metro stations, the closest being the Federal Center SW station. There are different ways to negotiate the 2.2 miles of the National Mall to the Lincoln Memorial. We suggest following Madison Drive on the right side of center. This takes you past the Ulysses S. Grant Memorial, then the massive Washington Monument which, when completed in 1885, was the tallest structure in the world. (That record was quickly quashed by the French who built the Eiffel Tower five years later.)

You then pass the new National WWII Memorial and the unobtrusive Vietnam Veterans Memorial, ending at the stately Lincoln Memorial where the 16th president still sits austerely on his big chair.

On this route you may encounter crowded spots, but there is generally enough space to be able to easily detour around any such human obstructions.

At the Lincoln Memorial, bear left towards the Potomac River and the Arlington Memorial Bridge. Cross the Potomac on this bridge, which has wide pedestrian and cyclist paths down both sides.

Across the river you are now in Arlington, Virginia. Congratulations! You have escaped the sightseers and joined the world of Washington's on-foot exercisers. You have some choices at this point. You can continue straight ahead to Arlington Cemetery if you wish; but we would not recommend that as a running place. Rather, in our next route, we shall take you to a good wind-down lunch spot from which you can conveniently access the Cemetery afterwards. Alternatively, you could head downstream on the Mount Vernon Trail, but that is longer and we shall cover that in our third route. For this first route, head upstream on the Mount Vernon Trail. You have to cross a couple of traffic lanes to get onto the trail, but that is not particularly difficult. The next part of the route is very pleasant, with scenic views of the Potomac throughout.

---

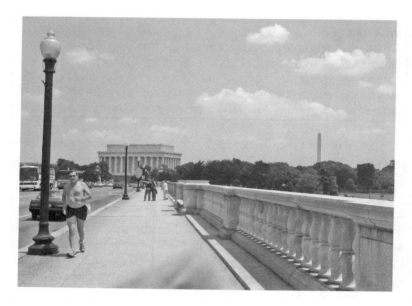

### Arlington Memorial Bridge

Pass the pedestrian bridge to Theodore Roosevelt Island, which is a 90-acre nature reserve, well worth seeing, but not a good running environment. Shortly afterwards, the path splits. Take the left-hand, wider path that leads to a footbridge over the George Washington Memorial Parkway. The trail off that bridge brings you out near the Key Bridge Marriott hotel, at the intersection of Lee Highway and Lynn Street in Rosslyn.

If you need a restroom or water fountain, both are located one block along Lee Highway at Fort Myer Drive, under the road overpass. If you have had enough on-foot activity and want to catch the Metro elsewhere, the Metro station is in Moore Street, between Lynn Street and Fort Myer Drive.

We recommend, however, that you head northwards up Lynn Street and cross the river via the sidewalk of the Francis Scott Key Bridge, named after the local revolutionary patriot and lyricist of the Star-Spangled Banner. This takes you to historic and action-filled Georgetown, which was established in 1751, over 40 years before Washington, DC.

While there are various things you may want to do in Georgetown, we suggest you first take this opportunity to see the Chesapeake and Ohio (C&O) Canal, continuing to get some on-foot exercise.

At the Georgetown end of the Key Bridge, on M Street, take a hard right down a footpath to the C&O Canal Towpath.

The C&O Canal is an amazing historical relic. It stretches 184 miles from Cumberland, Maryland to its downstream endpoint here in Georgetown. It took 22 years to build, from 1828 to its opening in 1850. It was designed for transporting all types of goods, via mule-towed barges. Unfortunately, its construction happened to coincide with the emergence of the railroad industry—the Baltimore and Ohio Railroad started construction the same year as the canal. Hence, somewhat obviously in retrospect, the canal ended up being obsolete before it opened. Clearly some investors backed the wrong horse (mule?) in financing this project!

Nevertheless, the canal did operate for 74 years and is now preserved as a National Historic Park. For hikers and other on-foot exercisers it represents a great opportunity since its towpath, designed for those poor mules, is still there. For runners, conditions up the towpath are highly variable, but the last piece down here in Georgetown is a real gem and not to be missed.

Today, the National Park Service operates canal boat tourist rides, complete with real mules and handlers in period costume. So you might even be treated to that spectacle when on-foot here. Apart from being careful where you tread, you will not find these activities an impediment to your on-foot exercising, since the towpath is in excellent condition for running, jogging, or walking.

We suggest following the canal downstream to Thomas Jefferson Street, less than a mile from Rosslyn. You then have some choices as to where to head:

- If you are staying in Georgetown or would like to see it, turn left and head up to M Street, the center of Georgetown life;
- If you want to have a pleasant wind-down break on the Potomac bank, head right to Washington Harbour (yes, it really is spelt that way);
- If you want to continue straight back to your downtown hotel, also head right but keep going east rather than stopping at Washington Harbour.

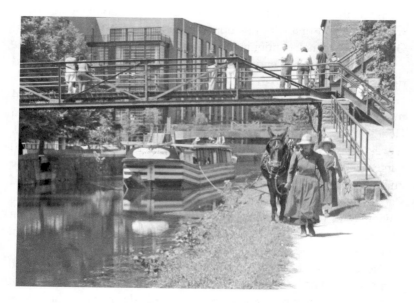

**Mule-Towed Barges on the C&O Canal**

If you decide to explore Georgetown, sights include:
- Alexander Graham Bell's laboratory (3414 Volta Place);
- The Oak Hill Cemetery, final resting place of many famous Americans (30th and R);
- Old Stone House, built in 1765 and thought to be the oldest standing building in Washington (3051 M);
- Dumbarton Oaks, where FDR hosted the conference that led to the United Nations Charter (1703 32nd); and
- Houses of many well-known former residents, including the Kennedys and Elizabeth Taylor.

Washington Harbour is a particularly pleasant place for winding down from a little on-foot exercise. You can grab a beer or have a good meal, in an outdoor environment where people in running gear fit in just fine. There are several restaurant/bar choices at Washington Harbour, including Tony and Joe's Seafood Place, Sequoia, and Nick's Riverside Grill. Regardless of your choice, given good weather, you will experience an excellent riverside environment.

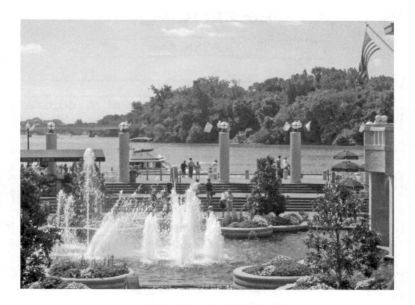

**Washington Harbour**

You can then either head back north to Georgetown proper, head eastward to the Foggy Bottom Metro station at L Street and 23$^{rd}$ Street, or follow the pedestrian trail down this side of the river, past the Watergate complex (remember what happened there?) and the JFK Theatre for the Performing Arts, back to the Lincoln Memorial.

Wherever you choose to go from here, we hope you will find this outing an enjoyable introduction to Washington on foot.

# Potomac Parks and Arlington

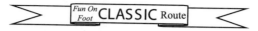

| Distance | 8.0 miles |
|---|---|
| Comfort | Excellent underfoot conditions on dedicated pedestrian/bicycle trails most of the way. Plenty of on-foot exercisers around but crowds are unlikely to be a problem. OK for inline skating. |
| Attractions | Pass the Washington Monument and the Jefferson, FDR, and Lincoln Memorials. Follow wide, attractive trails along the Potomac and in adjacent parks. These are popular on-foot exercising venues with Washington locals. |
| Convenience | Start near the Washington Monument, within easy walking distance of hotels in the Federal Triangle or L'Enfant Plaza vicinities, or take the Metro to Smithsonian (Blue and Orange Lines) or L'Enfant Plaza (Green and Yellow Lines). End at Courthouse Road in Arlington at a Metro Orange line Metro station. |
| Destination | The Courthouse Road area in Arlington, with several good pubs and restaurants for winding down, and convenient access to the Iwo Jima Memorial and Arlington National Cemetery for subsequent sightseeing. Metro stations are handy. |

In this route we focus more on pleasant runnable terrain and escape from sightseers, without getting very far away from the heart of DC. As always, you might want to keep all these ideas together or pull them apart and use them to construct your own favorite route.

The route starts on the National Mall at the Washington Monument. You pass by some other major monuments, generally bypassing the meandering sightseers. You experience some of the great on-foot trails on the Potomac, used extensively by the locals. Finally, we tack on a short stretch that brings you to a great restaurant/bar area, a short walk from the Iwo Jima Memorial and Arlington Cemetery.

To get started, find the Washington Monument. This is easy since it is so prominent. The closest Metro station is Smithsonian. Head south

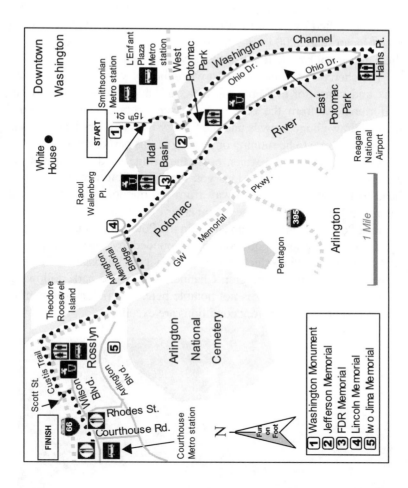

down 15<sup>th</sup> street, which becomes Raoul Wallenberg Place, dedicated to the famed Swedish industrialist-diplomat-humanitarian credited with saving a massive number of Jewish lives in World War II.

This brings you to the Tidal Basin and the Thomas Jefferson Memorial, which honors the nation's one and only really brilliant president. At a gathering of Nobel Peace Prize winners in the White House, President Kennedy is reported as declaring, "You are the greatest assembly of talent in the White House since Thomas Jefferson dined here alone."

This is also the location of the famous cherry trees—more than 3,000 of them—gifted by Japan in 1912 (following a failed attempt in 1910 when Japan sent 2,000 trees but the Agriculture Department destroyed them all for not having first had the necessary shots).

The cherry trees look their best when they bloom their magnificent pink and white for a couple of weeks in late March to early April. Unfortunately, from the on-foot exerciser's perspective, this nature display draws huge crowds and the Cherry Blossom Festival. This is not the best time to be running or jogging in this part of town.

When you reach the water, cross the bridge heading towards the Jefferson Memorial. This brings you into West Potomac Park. Then head to the left (southeast), away from the memorial and under the Interstate 395 highway bridges. You enter East Potomac Park.

East Potomac Park is on an island in the Potomac, occupied mainly by an 18-hole public golf course surrounded by various types of recreation areas. You effectively circumnavigate this island. Proceed along the northern (Washington Channel) side of the park, following Ohio Drive. The scenery is not notable here, but the environment is very pleasant and the on-foot conditions are excellent.

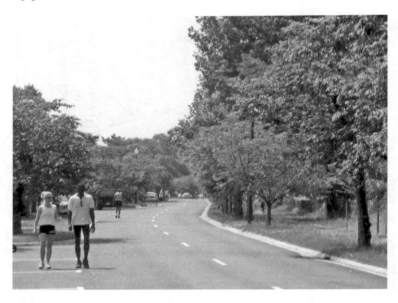

**East Potomac Park—Locals' Favorite On-foot Venue**

There is a sidewalk for part of the way and then you have a choice of using the road surface, the grass, or the path along the water, if it is not flooded. Running on the edge of the road is generally OK. While there is the occasional motor vehicle, on a nice day you will probably be sharing the route with more runners, walkers, cyclists, and inline skaters than motorists.

In summer, the lower half of the island is closed to motorists in late afternoon and evening on Saturdays, Sundays, and holidays.

At the southeastern end of the island, Hains Point, keep following the road which steers you around to head northwest along the Potomac River upstream. There are restrooms near Hains Point and also further up the river. You pass Ronald Reagan Washington National Airport on the opposite bank and, if the wind is right, get to observe at first hand the challenge faced by pilots as they fly down the river then have to negotiate a quick, sharp turn before dropping onto the runway. (They are barred from flying over the Federal Triangle area.)

After crossing under the highway bridges again, you re-enter West Potomac Park and see the Jefferson Memorial. You have traveled about 3.4 miles through the Potomac Parks. Unless you particularly want to visit the memorial, keep bearing left and cross the short Inlet Bridge, which takes you to Franklin Delano Roosevelt Memorial Park. If you have not seen the FDR Memorial before, we suggest you keep to the right-hand side that allows you to jog or walk straight through the memorial. This is a very tasteful memorial with more emphasis on space, flowing water, trees, and FDR's brilliant quotations than on marble construction as with some of the other memorials. If you do not want to traverse the memorial, bear left, keeping on the Potomac bank. Either way, you should end up back on the river. Continue one mile, close to the Lincoln Memorial. Unless you want to drop in to see that memorial, keep nearer the river and follow the road up to the eastern end of the Arlington Memorial Bridge.

You are now, for a while, retracing part of our first route. Cross the Potomac on the Arlington Memorial Bridge and take the Mount Vernon Trail northward or upstream. Follow our first route to Rosslyn, at the intersection of Lynn Street and Lee Highway.

If you want to end your run in Rosslyn, there are a few fast food places, a few hotel bars, and a Metro station in Moore Street (one block west of Lynn). However, there is nothing outstanding here in the food and beverage department. We therefore recommend you continue on-foot another 0.8 mile to a much more satisfying destination, just one stop further up the Metro Orange Line, where eating and drinking establishments are much superior.

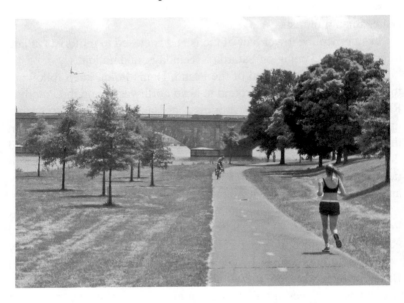

**Mount Vernon Trail on the Arlington Side of the Potomac**

The most efficient way there is to follow the Lee Highway sidewalk past the Marriott Hotel. This leads you to the Martha Custis Trail, a bicycle trail that connects four miles further on with the 45-mile-long Washington and Old Dominion (W&OD) Trail. The latter trail, which extends through Northern Virginia following an old railroad route as far as Purcellville, is really more suitable for cycling than on-foot exercise, so we do not propose going out there.

The Custis Trail follows Interstate 66. We suggest going only as far as Scott Street, where you can cross the highway via an overpass, then track westward via Quinn Street and Wilson Boulevard to the Rhodeside Grill at Rhodes Street and Wilson.

The Rhodeside Grill is a good choice for a wind-down break, especially if you want to then see Arlington's main memorials.

There are also several interesting wind-down options just a block further up Wilson Boulevard, in the Courthouse Road vicinity. They are ideal if you intend to catch the Metro immediately afterwards. Some places have a Sunday brunch and a couple of them have a Saturday brunch as well. Our hearts (and stomachs) found post-run satisfaction at Ireland's Four Courts pub at Wilson and Courthouse. This is a nicely decorated traditional Irish pub with excellent food and an extensive beer menu. You can catch the Metro at the Courthouse Station a short distance up Wilson.

If you want to see Arlington's unforgettable monuments, here are the directions. From the Rhodeside Grill, take Rhodes Street southward, cross the Arlington Boulevard highway, then follow the street on the highway's southern edge eastward. This brings you to the very impressive Iwo Jima Memorial, which is dedicated to all U.S. Marines who gave their lives in defense of the nation.

From this memorial, you can easily trek southward a short distance to Arlington National Cemetery, pay your respects to the nation's heroes, and catch the Metro home from the cemetery's Metro station.

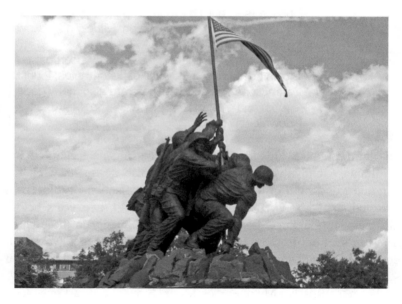

**The Iwo Jima Memorial**

# Mount Vernon Trail to Alexandria

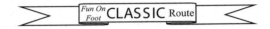

| Distance | 10.0 miles |
|---|---|
| Comfort | Excellent on-foot conditions on a dedicated pedestrian/bicycle trail. There are plenty of cyclists and some runners and walkers. Be sure to carry some water. OK for inline skating. |
| Attractions | Follow the beautiful Potomac River past some of the main national capital monuments, Reagan National Airport, and some less inhabited terrain, to a very attractive old town with many historic sights and activities. |
| Convenience | Start at Rosslyn, which is less than a mile on-foot from Georgetown and on the Metro Blue and Orange Lines. Alternatively, you can pick up the trail at the Arlington end of the Arlington Memorial Bridge, one-to-two miles from most downtown hotels (see our first route for directions). End at the King Street Metro station (Blue and Yellow Lines) in Alexandria. |
| Destination | Old Town Alexandria, the oldest incorporated town in this region. It is full of historic sites, tourist attractions and shops. There are also many good pubs and restaurants. Catch the Metro back downtown. |

Our third route is a little longer but fits all our route-selection criteria admirably. It involves following the Potomac downstream on the Virginia side to the historic and enjoyable destination of Old Town Alexandria. Alexandria was established in 1749, two years before Georgetown, making it the oldest formal community in these parts. You can start out from anywhere in the Potomac-Georgetown region covered in our previous routes, but we shall describe the route as if you started from the Rosslyn Metro station.

From the Rosslyn Metro exit on Moore Street, head east one block and north two blocks to the intersection of Lynn Street and Lee Highway. Take the paved path down towards the river, following the sign to the Mount Vernon Trail. Take that trail southbound. If you started at the

Lincoln Monument, you can pick up the same trail after crossing the Arlington Memorial Bridge.

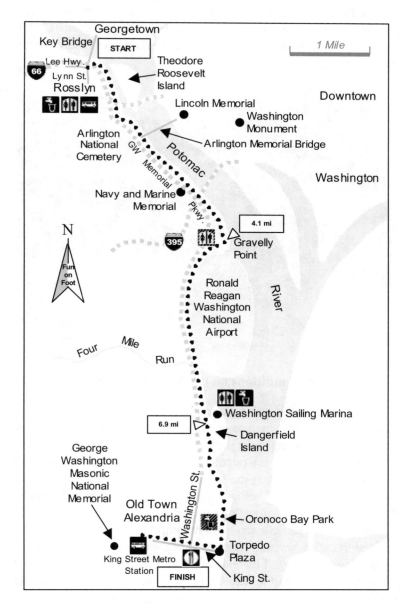

This is an excellent trail. You do not need to cross a trafficked street for roughly 7.5 miles, until you reach Alexandria. The trail is paved and is shared by pedestrians and cyclists. Your biggest comfort concern, on a busy summer weekend day, might be too many cyclists. Take comfort, though, from the signs that state clearly that cyclists must give way to pedestrians.

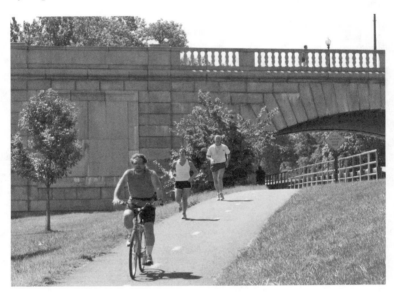

**Typical Conditions on the Mount Vernon Trail**

At 2.9 miles from Rosslyn, you pass the Navy and Marine Memorial, dedicated in 1934 to Americans who served at sea. Another 1.2 miles further on, after passing under the Interstate 395 road bridges, you come to Gravelly Point. This is a popular spot for locals. Its main value is as a parking lot for accessing the Mount Vernon Trail, but it also has the fascinating attraction of being at the northern end of Ronald Reagan Washington National Airport's main runway.

That airport's name is too big a mouthful for everyday use. While we used to call it *National Airport*, with respect for *the Gipper* I now call it *Reagan Airport*. I have no doubt that this name will soon be its popular handle, given the way we have readily adopted the monikers *JFK*, *O'Hare*, *Dulles*, and *Logan* for some other famous airports.

One of the attractions of Gravelly Point is the novel experience of having large aircraft pass a couple of hundred feet over your head while either landing or taking off at Reagan. This is not the sort of thing most people would spend the afternoon doing, but one or two such aircraft events mid-route definitely help take a runner's mind off the body's other current concerns, such as aching muscles and joints. Furthermore, Gravelly Point offers one of the few restroom stops on this route.

After Gravelly Point, the trail diverts away from the river in order to bypass Reagan Airport. The scenery therefore becomes more one of cars, people, planes, and trains than a nature scene. However, the planners have done an excellent job in keeping the trail pleasant and free from any direct vehicle encounters.

After Reagan Airport you come to an interesting trail intersection. The Four Mile Run trail heads westward away from the river here. This trail connects with the 45-mile-long Washington and Old Dominion (W&OD) trail; an interesting route for cyclists but not so exciting for runners, unless you happen to live somewhere near it. For now, we suggest keeping on the Mount Vernon Trail southbound.

At 2.8 miles from Gravelly Point, you intersect the access road to the Dangerfield Island sporting and recreation area (no longer an island) and the Washington Sailing Marina. If you need a break by now, there are restrooms, water, and even a restaurant here. When Nola and I did this run on a fairly hot day last summer, we really welcomed reaching this spot since we were running short of water and Alexandria was still some distance away.

At the southern end of the Dangerfield Island area, the trail splits. You should choose the option closest to the river, which is known as the Alexandria Waterfront Walk or the River Route. This trail has helpful signs identifying the several parks it traverses. While you are now following streets more so than before, there is little vehicular traffic to annoy you. By the time you reach Madison Street, the northern end of Oronoco Bay, conditions are becoming decidedly more urbanized, but in a pleasant way. There is even a water fountain right beside the trail at Madison Street—the first since leaving Rosslyn.

After passing City Marina, almost two miles from the Dangerfield Island access road, you reach Torpedo Plaza. This is effectively the heart of Old Town Alexandria. Alexandria started as a settlement in 1669 when Scotsman John Alexander purchased all the land here. Alexandria formally became a Virginia town in 1749, and was a major 18th century port. It is considered the primary home of George Washington (whose Mount Vernon estate is a few miles away to the south), revolutionary hero General Henry "Light Horse Harry" Lee, and his son, General Robert E. Lee, commander in chief of the Confederate army.

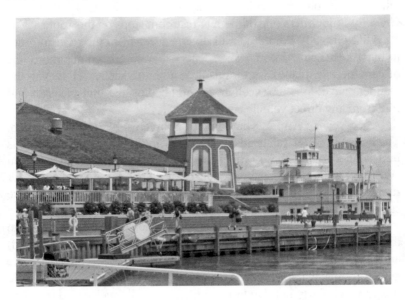

**Torpedo Plaza, Old Town Alexandria**

The Torpedo Factory Art Center is a transformed 1920 munitions factory, which once produced MK-14 torpedoes. Now it houses artists' studios and workshops.

The Old Town's main activity is in or near King Street, which heads inland from Torpedo Plaza and eventually leads you to the King Street Metro station.

Driving and parking in Old Town Alexandria are nightmares. You will feel pretty good at this point if you are on foot and your only challenges are to find the most enjoyable places in this action-filled and history-filled town, and then catch the Metro home.

After Nola's and my hot day's run from Rosslyn, we badly needed and felt no guilt whatsoever in seeking out a good watering hole with food. We found two excellent Irish pubs, and did not skimp on the time spent in sampling them both. Pat Troy's Ireland's Own, at the corner of King Street and Pitt Street served a good brunch, good drinks, and generally brought us back to a feel-good state. It is authentically Irish, including corners honoring various personalities, the most significant (when we were there, at least) being Ronald Reagan's corner. Reagan visited here during his 1988 presidential campaign and clearly left his mark on the place. There was even live entertainment on a Saturday afternoon.

Murphy's, a block further up King Street, was at least as good. It has a lovely décor and a warm, cozy atmosphere. It also sports an enormous collection of police badges from around the nation. We fell into conversation with several locals and an Australian photographer doing a photo shoot for ads for the Guinness brewery. I ended up accepting a gratis Guinness resulting from the photo shoot since I was the only person involved who was not on duty. (I was definitely feeling good about fun-on-foot at this point!) We also had dinner at Murphy's that evening and can recommend the food.

There are several other restaurants in Old Town, some of which we have sampled, always with positive results. For example, we really enjoyed Tiffany Tavern, a small, friendly place with swinging bluegrass music. There are also several historic sites in Old Town, with a sign-posted walking tour that links them.

The King Street Metro station is 1.2 miles up King Street from Torpedo Plaza. On weekends there is a free shuttle bus along King Street, but as an on-foot aficionado that probably does not matter to you.

Just beyond the Metro station, you can see the imposing George Washington Masonic National Memorial. There are free tours daily. This site, Shuter's Hill, is also where Orville Wright first demonstrated his aircraft to the Federal government in 1909. If you have time before catching the Metro, it is well worth a visit.

# Rock Creek Park to Georgetown

| | |
|---|---|
| **Distance** | 6.0 miles |
| **Comfort** | Good running and jogging conditions, except for a one-mile hiking stretch in Soapstone Valley. Expect other pedestrians around, except Soapstone Valley where you might be alone. (You can bypass that part if you wish.) Crowds are unlikely to be a problem. The route is mostly shady and generally flat. Not suitable for inline skating. |
| **Attractions** | Widely varied terrain, much of it of a wilderness nature. Escape from the crowds, vehicles, and city scene. Pass the Peirce Mill, National Zoo, and Mount Zion Cemetery, and end near Georgetown's many tourist attractions. |
| **Convenience** | Start at the Van Ness-UDC Metro station on the Red Line, which services, among other destinations, Bethesda, Woodley Park, Dupont Circle, and downtown Washington. Finish in Georgetown, within easy walking distance of Rosslyn, Foggy Bottom, and Dupont Circle precincts, and handy to Blue and Orange Line Metro stations. |
| **Destination** | Historic and character-rich Georgetown, with many sights to see, including Alexander Graham Bell's Laboratory and the 1765-vintage Old Stone House. There are many good pubs and restaurants for winding down. |

Our next route aims to satisfy the on-foot exerciser's needs for some wilderness and escape from people, without ever leaving DC. It centers on Rock Creek Park, one of Washington's greatest assets. Occupying 1,775 acres, it is more than twice the size of New York's Central Park and consumes 4.5% of the entire land area of the District of Columbia. Interesting wildlife, especially bird life, can be found throughout the widely varied terrain. In much of the park, no civilization can be seen, so one can easily forget one is, in fact, in the middle of Washington. Established in 1890, its natural state has been preserved relatively unscathed, except for the inevitable roads that make their way through and across it and a few developments such as the National Zoological Park.

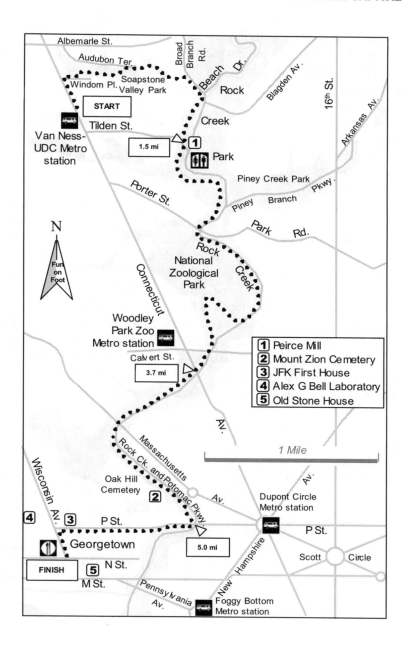

Albemarle St.

Audubon Ter.

Broad Branch Rd.

Beach Dr.

Windom Pl. Soapstone Valley Park

Rock

Blagden Av.

16th St.

Arkansas Av.

**START**

Tilden St.

Creek

1.5 mi

Van Ness-UDC Metro station

1 Park

Piney Creek Park

Porter St.

Piney Branch Pkwy.

Park Rd.

N

Fun on Foot

Rock Creek

Connecticut

National Zoological Park

Woodley Park Zoo Metro station

Calvert St.

3.7 mi

1 Peirce Mill
2 Mount Zion Cemetery
3 JFK First House
4 Alex G Bell Laboratory
5 Old Stone House

Av.

1 Mile

Massachusetts

Rock Ck. and Potomac Pkwy.

Av.

Dupont Circle Metro station

Wisconsin Av.

Oak Hill Cemetery

2

4 3 P St.

Georgetown

FINISH

5 N St.

M St.

Pennsylvania Av.

New Hampshire

P St.

Scott Circle

Foggy Bottom Metro station

5.0 mi

While there are many options for traversing the park on foot, the best ones from the comfort and convenience perspectives are unquestionably in the southern part of the park. We put together a six-mile route which is mainly within the park but which tacks on a very interesting starting segment and a compelling destination in historic and lively Georgetown.

Start at the Van Ness-UDC Red Line Metro station. There are different ways to get from this Metro station onto the main trail in Rock Creek Park. We shall recommend a particularly awesome one. (It does come with a few caveats—I shall mention some other options without the caveats later.)

Take the Metro station exit on the east side of Connecticut Avenue, then head north up Connecticut less than 200 yards to Windom Place. Turn right. After about 100 yards, on the left, you come to a gap in the fence giving access to an obscure little trailhead. There is a small sign declaring the Soapstone Valley Trail, 0.9 mile to Rock Creek, trail maintained by the Potomac Appalachian Trail Club.

Enter the trail and take the path heading off hard right. Within no more than another 100 yards you are in a new world that you would never have imagined existed. You are in the midst of a lush rainforest with no signs or sounds of civilization—just a little-used path following the course of a babbling stream. True! You have traveled less than a quarter mile from getting off a Metro train on one of Washington's busiest avenues, and you now feel you have been magically teleported to a wilderness scene in a different region, state, country, ...maybe planet.

This feeling stays with you as you follow the trail along the creek, crossing the creek several times on stepping-stones. When we were there, there were no people anywhere and no signs that anyone had been there any time in recent history. Generally the under-foot conditions are sound, but it is no walk in the park. Let us be quite clear—this is not a run—it is a backwoods hike. In spots, the going gets a little steep and you face a real possibility of slipping off a rock into a shallow stream if you are not careful. Seasoned hikers will love this trail. Street bound city dwellers might have reservations, but Nola and I both felt strongly that the benefits greatly outweighed the reservations.

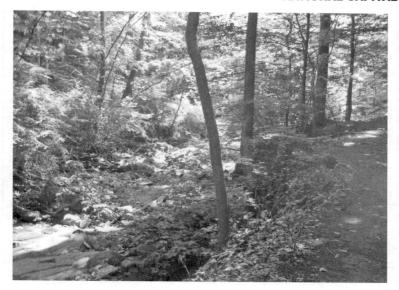

**Soapstone Valley—Virgin Rainforest Hidden Deep within the Urban Jungle**

After 0.4 mile, the trail makes its first return to civilization at the south end of Audubon Terrace, a lovely hidden residential street. You quickly find, however, a new entrance to the continuation of the trail to your right. The going from here on is a little better than the first part. After another 0.4 mile the trail comes out abruptly on a lightly-to-moderately trafficked two-lane road called Broad Branch Road. Follow this road to the right. This is probably the least pleasant part of the whole route since there is no sidewalk and there *is* some vehicle traffic.

After about 150 yards you reach the intersection of Broad Branch Road and Beach Drive. Keep to the right-hand side of the creek—do not take Beach Drive. Enter an unnamed street with a parking lot adjacent. The street, as such, abruptly ends with a barrier to preclude further progress by vehicles. This automobile-free track then morphs into a paved bike trail. This is the inauspicious start of the Rock Creek bike trail, which continues from here right down to the Lincoln Memorial. You have traveled 1.3 miles from the Metro station.

---

**VARIATION**

There are some alternatives to traversing Soapstone Valley Park. You might prefer these if you don't like off-road hiking terrain or are concerned about the solitude in that park when you are out unaccompanied. One option, which bypasses the toughest part of the hiking terrain, is to continue up Connecticut Avenue past Windom Place to Albemarle Street. Take Albemarle to 29th Street to Audubon Terrace, and then pick up the final (easier) part of the Soapstone Valley Trail at the eastern end of Audubon. Another alternative, which cuts out the backwoods stretch entirely, is to head southward on Connecticut from the Metro station to Tilden Street. Tilden takes you to the Peirce Mill where you intersect the paved pedestrian/bike trail.

---

The hiking and road-walking parts of this route are now over, and you can run or jog the rest if you wish. The Rock Creek Trail is generally very pleasant. There is a paved path all the way and also unpaved walking side paths much of the way. The only somewhat unpleasant aspect of this trail is that, in parts, it runs adjacent to the busy Rock Creek and Potomac Parkway.

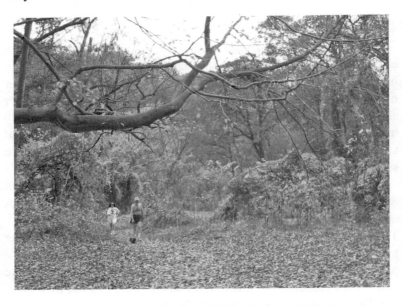

**Rock Creek Trail in Fall—Hard to Believe This is in the Middle of DC**

---

After 0.2 mile, you pass the well-preserved Peirce Mill, built in 1827. This was one of eight water-driven grain-grinding mills originally on Rock Creek. It operated commercially until 1897. It was restored to operation in 1936 and was in working order until 1993. Efforts continue to restore it to operation yet again.

Continue along the trail to the National Zoological Park. If you are serious about your on-foot exercise, you probably don't want to drop into the zoo right now. However, you might want to come back here another time to see the giant pandas gifted by the People's Republic of China in 2000. Interestingly, the 160-acre zoo property was landscaped originally by none other than Frederick Law Olmsted—the very same man who was responsible for New York's Central Park and Boston's Emerald Necklace. Mr. Olmsted truly left his mark on the U.S. urban scene in a big way!

At the zoo, the trail parts company with the noisy Parkway for half a mile. The trail follows the creek, largely under shady trees, which make for very pleasant conditions. Eventually you rejoin the Parkway. After a further 0.2 mile, near the Connecticut Avenue high-level arch bridge, there is a Parkway exit with a pedestrian sidewalk if you want to leave the park. That is useful if you are staying in the Connecticut/Calvert area, but otherwise we suggest you continue on.

After a couple more high-level bridges you come to the Mount Zion cemetery on the western bank. Cross the creek via a footbridge here. Proceed to the next overhead road crossing, where there is also a Parkway exit ramp. This is 1.3 miles past Connecticut Avenue. Walk up the edge of that ramp, which brings you to P Street in Georgetown.

Georgetown is a fine destination for an on-foot outing. Follow P Street westbound to Wisconsin Avenue, passing John and Jackie Kennedy's original Georgetown residence at 3271 P Street. Turn left into Wisconsin Avenue and you are now presented with a range of sightseeing, eating, drinking, and shopping choices. For some sightseeing pointers, see our National Mall and the Potomac route description.

The restaurants and pubs are mainly on Wisconsin Avenue or M Street. In the pub-restaurant category, we can strongly recommend Martin's Tavern, in Wisconsin at N Street, a mile from where you left Rock Creek. This is a classy Irish pub with great food, but it is not so pretentious that you feel unwelcome dropping in there in your running gear. I can attest that the clam chowder and the Maryland crab cakes are excellent. Martin's has hosted several Presidents, including John Kennedy, Harry Truman, Lyndon Johnson and Richard Nixon.

Getting to the Metro involves a roughly 15-minute walk, either along P Street to Dupont Circle or M Street and Pennsylvania Avenue to Foggy Bottom.

---

**VARIATIONS**

Should you not want to end your route at Georgetown, there are some alternative terminations. One is to not exit the trail at P Street, but continue down the creek to the Lincoln Memorial and the National Mall. Another option is to exit at P Street but, rather than go west into Georgetown, go east towards Dupont Circle. There are many restaurants around P and 21st or a little further south at M and 21st. Our favorite is the Sign of the Whale Pub on M Street.

---

# Other Ideas

There are other good running routes around Washington DC, some of which are simply extensions or variants of what we have already described.

From Alexandria, you can follow the **Mount Vernon Trail** southward to the Mount Vernon Estate. From Rosslyn you can follow the **Martha Custis Trail** to the 45-mile-long Washington and Old Dominion (W&OD) Trail. While this is something of a marathon, you can get to some of the Orange Line Metro stations quite easily from the Custis Trail.

Alternatively, you could follow the **C&O Canal towpath** upstream, starting from Georgetown. Unfortunately, since there is no Metro service in that direction, it is a challenge to build a circle route up that way.

In Rock Creek Park, you can also extend your travel on the **Rock Creek Trail** both northward and (as we already mentioned) southward. The northward extension is best on Saturday, Sunday, or a holiday when Beach Drive is closed to vehicle traffic from Military Road to Broad Branch Road. The latter point is at the start of the paved trail we used in our Rock Creek route. One issue you have to deal with is how to get to or from Military Road, since there is not a very convenient Metro station.

Another option is to simply run or walk around the downtown DC streets, such as in the **National Mall/Federal Triangle** area, soaking in the sights on the way. This is a fine idea from the attractions, convenience, and destination perspectives, since there are many things to see, plenty of convenient Metro stations, and many fine eating and drinking establishments at which to terminate. Comfort could be an issue owing to sightseer crowds getting in your way, but you can avoid them by starting early. I'll leave it as an exercise to the reader to devise some interesting routes along those lines.

\* \* \* \*

It is time to wind up our visit to the nation's capital and move on to other parts of the country. My parting message for this city: Follow the examples of Jimmy Carter, the Presidents Bush, and Bill Clinton. Get out on foot regularly and, when in DC, use the on-foot approach as a way to soak in the sights and escape the stress. And, above all, enjoy it!

# 6

# Peach City

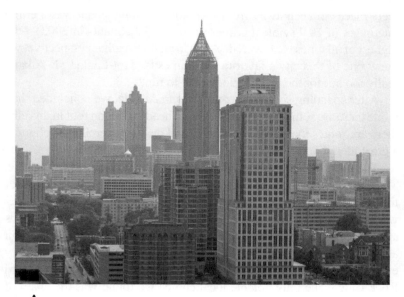

Atlanta, Georgia, is a comparatively young city, starting as a railroad hub in 1836. Its first major place in history relates to the Civil War, having been attacked, evacuated, and burned to the ground by the Union forces in 1864. The fall of Atlanta is seen by many as the most critical point in the war, bolstering the confidence of the North, and leading to the re-election of Abraham Lincoln and the eventual surrender of the Confederates. Atlanta was also the birthplace of Martin Luther King, Jr. and the nerve center of the civil rights movements of the 1950s and 1960s.

Atlanta does not instantly leap into most people's minds as a great city in which to be out on-foot. Nevertheless, it is such a prominent city we decided to consider it.

In our initial research, on the positive side, we found some strong recommendations. In particular, *Runner's World* ranked Atlanta as number 7 in its 2002 "10 Best Running Cities" in the United States.[1] Even more surprisingly, Atlanta and Boston were the only cities, from the set we toured, to make this top 10. Mike Cosentino's excellent book, *Atlanta Running Guide*,[2] further declared that 25% of the population consider themselves to be runners or joggers.

On the negative side, we had heard opinions from various present or past area residents that downtown Atlanta and much of its surrounds were places to keep away from. Another warning signal was a crime rate index of 19.7 (violent crimes per 1,000 inhabitants in 2003)—the highest of all cities we covered. Also, from the weather perspective, we knew one of this city's favorite nicknames is "Hot-Lanta." Is Atlanta really too hot for the average Joe or Jill to run?

After spending some time ourselves in Atlanta, we concluded that, while there are some qualifications about heading out on foot in this city, there are routes that meet our criteria and on-foot exercise is definitely a great idea if you are in the area.

The main letdown is *downtown* Atlanta, which is a pretty dull place. There are several large hotels that attract conventions. Were it not for that, the city would be dead at night and nothing more than an office-worker enclave in the daytime. The most exciting tourist attractions are the CNN Center and the World of Coca-Cola. The restaurant and pub choices are OK but limited. The high points of our culinary experiences were Benihana's (we always love Benihana's) and the Hard Rock Café. The only notable local choice we found was the chain of Mick's restaurant/pubs.

The truth is that most good things about Atlanta are quite a way from downtown. All the night action, for example, is in the northern suburbs, such as Buckhead. Also, when people get enthusiastic about running in Atlanta, you will generally find they are thinking about places like Stone Mountain, a superb spot with excellent jogging/running trails and plenty of attractions. However, Stone Mountain is 16 miles from the city, has two hotels (both up-market), and has virtually no public transit. One generally needs to drive through a lot of congested traffic to get there.

---

1      See: http://www.runnersworld.com/article/0,5033,s6-188-0-0-1199-1-4X7-3,00.html

2      Peachtree Publishers Ltd., Atlanta GA, 2003.

Nevertheless, I figured I would put the city's core custodians to the test. I walked into the city information office downtown and asked them for their recommendations as to "running trails" or "jogging trails" convenient to downtown. I know I have a funny accent (a slightly Bostonized and Canadianized Australian accent) but was still surprised at the difficulty I had in getting these people to understand what I was asking. They were very friendly and keen to help, but it soon became pretty clear they had never had anyone ask for either of these things before. Eventually one young woman caught on, and offered helpfully that she had once seen someone running in Olympic/Centennial Park. However, that was it. They had nothing useful to offer. [3]

Undaunted, we pushed on, armed with suggestions from our Atlanta friends and the *Atlanta Running Guide*. We ended up with two routes that satisfy our criteria of comfort, attractions, convenience, and destination. There are definitely some opportunities for enjoyable on-foot exercise here.

I said earlier that there were some qualifications about on-foot exercise in Atlanta—they mainly relate to comfort. First, the safety angle: Remain astute, especially after dark and anywhere south of Interstate 20 at any time. An arguably bigger comfort concern is the weather. In summer, Atlanta *does* tend to be hot (the average maximum exceeds 80 degrees June through September), humid, and susceptible to thunderstorms. October through May are generally nice months for outdoor exercise. It rains roughly one day in three year-round, much the same as more northerly east-coast cities.

Also, while you will see the occasional other on-foot exerciser around, there are not a lot of them near downtown.

Driving in Atlanta tends to be a nightmare because of the massive traffic jams that often tie up the main arteries, especially the intertwining Interstate 75 and 85 highway systems. The city does not have a reputation for pedestrian friendliness, ever since the 1949 death of *Gone with the Wind* author Margaret Mitchell, struck by an automobile while crossing Peachtree Street. However, in our experience, the highway traffic pressures do not spread into the ordinary streets. On any routes that we traversed, while there was certainly traffic around, vehicles never became a particular concern to us.

---

3        In fact, some people do run in Olympic/Centennial Park, but it is a short loop with little appeal.

Atlanta does have a very good public transit system. The MARTA has a lengthy north-south subway line and a shorter east-west line, with a good network of connecting buses. (Unfortunately there is no subway or other fast transit to Stone Mountain.) The subway trains run frequently and are clean. The ticket machines have minds of their own, but that is not unique to this city.

We ended up selecting two on-foot routes in the corridor from downtown through Midtown to Buckhead, in which the vast majority of hotels are located. We hope you like them...

| Route | Distance |
|---|---|
| 1.  Downtown to Buckhead via Peachtree | 7.6 miles |
| 2.  Piedmont Park and Vicinity | 4.5-to-8.1 miles |

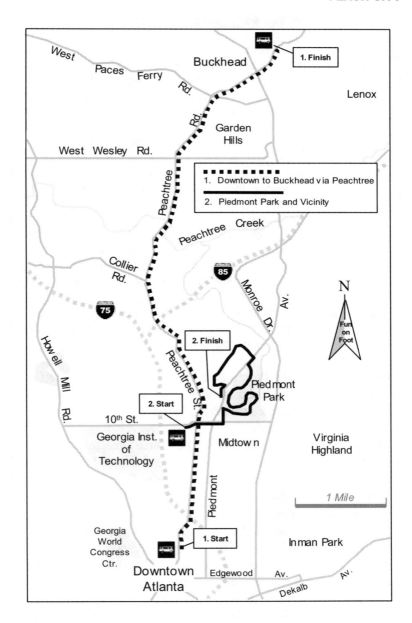

**Atlanta Routes**

# Downtown to Buckhead via Peachtree

| Distance | 7.6 miles |
|---|---|
| Comfort | The entire run is along good street sidewalks. It is relatively level. There is plenty of traffic but it does not impede the on-foot exerciser. There are food outlets on the way and some opportunities to bail out near subway stops. Expect to encounter other on-foot exercisers but not crowds. Questionable for inline skating. |
| Attractions | Touch the pulse of Atlanta life in the South's most famous thoroughfare. Follow the route of the world's largest 10K race and part of the Atlanta Marathon. |
| Convenience | Start downtown at the Peachtree Center, within easy walking distance of all downtown hotels, and at a station on the North-South MARTA line. End in Buckhead, at the Buckhead station on the North-South MARTA line. |
| Destination | Buckhead, with some excellent wind-down restaurant/bars, shops, and convenient transit back downtown. |

Atlanta, capital of the Peach State and located on Peachtree Creek, is a very peachy city. It hosts the Peach Bowl. It has a New Year Peach Drop, the Peachtree Center, and at least two-dozen streets with "Peachtree" in their names.

I think the best-known Peachtree is Peachtree Street that runs through Downtown and about four miles north. It then becomes Peachtree Road, which continues north several further miles to Buckhead and beyond. Peachtree Street is Atlanta's main drag.

For our first route, we therefore chose to cover from downtown, where most visitors stay, to Buckhead, where most of the action is, via Peachtree Street and Peachtree Road. If you are staying at a downtown hotel, this makes for a nice loop outing—do this route on-foot, sample Buckhead's offerings, and return downtown on the MARTA subway. You could do the route in reverse if you prefer.

This route satisfies all our criteria. Conditions are comfortable, including ample food, drink, and restroom opportunities at fast food outlets or other commercial establishments on the way.

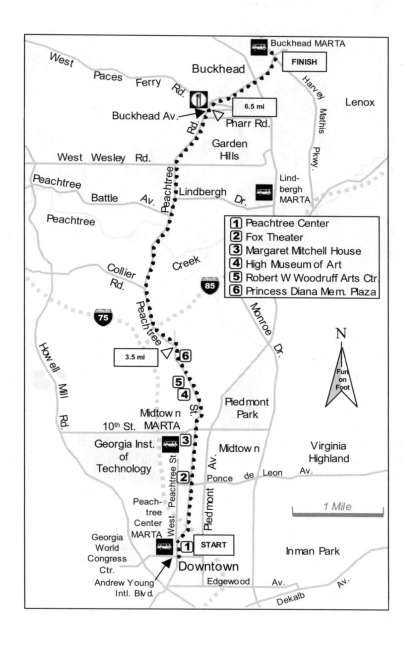

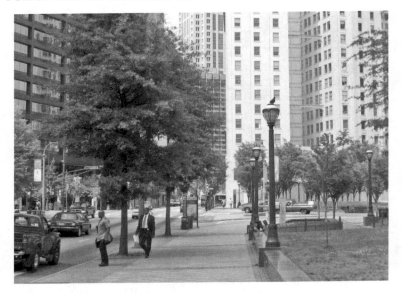

**Downtown Peachtree Street's Wide Sidewalk**

Start at the Peachtree Center, close to downtown hotels, at Peachtree Street and Andrew Young International Boulevard. Head northward on Peachtree Street. Even though you are in the middle of a busy city, the going is quite good. Peachtree Street has wide sidewalks and is typically not crowded.

At Baker Street, Peachtree Street splits into West Peachtree Street to the left and Peachtree Street to the right. Keep to Peachtree Street, which takes you over the Interstate 75 and 85 highways. At North Avenue, if you turned left it would take you to the Georgia Institute of Technology campus. We have done some running through the campus—it was reasonable but not sufficiently attractive for us to recommend a route there.

After Ponce de Leon Avenue, the numbered street system starts. Pass the classy Fox Theater, a National Historic Landmark, and continue up to 10th Street. The Margaret Mitchell House, complete with loads of *Gone with the Wind* memorabilia, is on the left. If you headed right here you would get to Piedmont Park, which we cover in our next route. Also, note that the rest of our route from here tracks (in the reverse direction) the course of the popular 10-kilometer Peachtree Road Race held every July 4.

Continue northward past the art museums between 15th and 16th Streets. A little further on, Peachtree Street re-merges with West Peachtree Street. Two blocks further on, Peachtree Road peels off to the left. Be sure to follow that road rather than West Peachtree Street, which quickly peters out.

Cross the Interstate 85 overpass and continue to Peachtree Creek. From downtown to this point the grade has been slightly downhill—not particularly steep. After the creek, the grade changes to slightly uphill but not steep enough to trouble the average on-foot exerciser.

---

**VARIATION**

Between Lindbergh Drive and Wesley Drive East there is an opportunity to divert away from the traffic and into the pleasant residential area of Garden Hills on the eastern side of Peachtree Road. There are some nice green strips through here. However, there are some substantial grades and the sidewalks are questionable and sometimes nonexistent. Therefore, this diversion is not for everyone and not our foremost recommendation.

---

On Peachtree Road there are several restaurant choices if you are ready for a break, especially north of Wesley Drive. However, we suggest you go on nearer to Buckhead, where you will also be close to the MARTA station for return travel.

For an interesting wind-down spot, we can recommend the Fado Irish Pub at Peachtree Road and Buckhead Avenue, just north of Pharr Road. Fado is now a chain of establishments, but this particular one is where it all started. Fado is Gaelic for "long ago," used, for example, for a storyteller to commence a tale. It is an interestingly decorated place, with great food, drinks, and atmosphere.

We have also sampled the Cheesecake Factory across the road from Fado, and found that to be an excellent all-round establishment.

After winding down at Fado or the Cheesecake Factory, you can then push on a further 1.1 miles along Peachtree to the Buckhead MARTA station, and ride in comfort back to downtown or Midtown.

# Piedmont Park and Vicinity

| Distance | 4.5-to-8.1 miles |
|---|---|
| Comfort | Pleasant running conditions, roughly half on dedicated pedestrian trails. Some following of sidewalks on suburban streets or busier roads. Expect to encounter other on-foot exercisers in daylight hours but not crowds. Not suitable in parts for inline skating. |
| Attractions | Experience Atlanta's largest and most pleasant urban park, plus some attractive nearby suburban neighborhoods. |
| Convenience | A loop in the Midtown area, north of downtown. Start at 10th Street and Peachtree Street, near the Midtown MARTA station on the North-South line. That line services downtown Atlanta, Buckhead, and other points north and south. You can travel here on-foot from downtown; add 1.4 miles each way and see our previous route for directions and conditions. We nominally finish at the Prince of Wales pub, but you can continue 0.8 miles to close the loop back to 10th Street and Peachtree. Total loop distance from the Midtown MARTA station is 5.5 miles and from downtown Atlanta is 8.1 miles. |
| Destination | Some good restaurant/pubs in the immediate vicinity, our favorite being the Prince of Wales English pub. Convenient transit to downtown, Buckhead, or other destinations on the MARTA line. |

Atlanta's largest and proudest city park is Piedmont Park, north of Midtown and just a couple of blocks east of Peachtree Street. It occupies about 190 acres, quite tiny compared with the city parks of New York, Philadelphia, and Washington, but attracting 2.5 million visitors annually nevertheless.

This land, originally farmland, was part of the site of the 1864 Battle at Peachtree Creek. A Confederate division dug in along its northern edge to repel the approach of the Union army under General Sherman. The land was then purchased in 1887 to build a horseracing track. It became the site of the 1895 Cotton States and International Exposition,

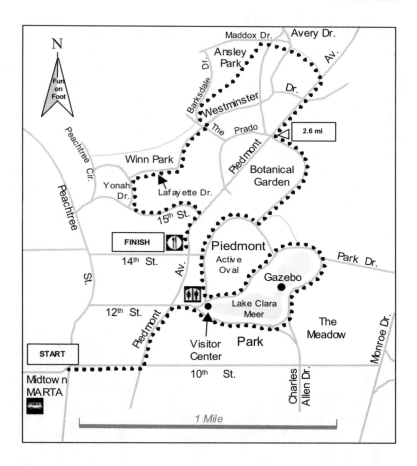

which included the first international showing of motion pictures. It was purchased by the city in 1904 for parkland purposes.

We shall assume a start at the corner of Peachtree Street and 10th Street. This is a short walk from Midtown. From downtown, you can run or walk up Peachtree Street (add about 1.4 miles) or take the MARTA to the Midtown Station and walk to the Peachtree intersection.

Follow 10th Street eastward two blocks to Piedmont Avenue, turn left, and enter Piedmont Park via the gate at 12th Street. You come to the park's Visitor Center—it has restrooms and a custodian, but not much that we could elicit in the way of information or even a map.

Bear right, following the road closest to the park's southern edge, with Lake Clara Meer on your left. By now you will be appreciating a valuable attribute of Piedmont Park—it is closed to automobiles.

You come to a road intersection, with the Meadow straight ahead. Both the lakes and the Meadow are suitable for running laps. We suggest doing a full lap (1.0 mile) around the lakes. You may wish to add on some more laps of the lakes or the Meadow, but our nominal route continues through the park, followed by some venturing into other parkland areas nearby.

In going around the lakes, the most scenic view is at the top end of the northern lake, where you are treated to a view of the lakes, the gazebo at their middle point, and Midtown high-rises in the background. After completely circumnavigating the lakes, you are back near the Visitor Center.

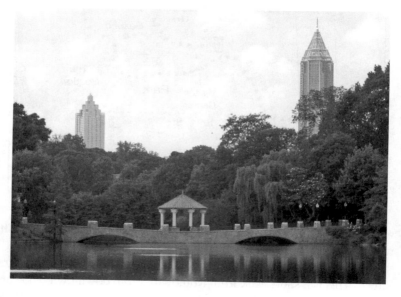

**Scenic Piedmont Park**

While Piedmont Park is very pleasant, it does not offer a very long on-foot route, so we decided to tack on some more interesting additions that include a mix of nearby residential areas and suburban parks.

We suggest heading north from the Visitor Center, around the sporting fields. Then, just before the tennis courts, take the path northwards that goes around the Atlanta Botanical Garden. It is a pleasant path with some trails off to the right into the woods, but the woods are not suitable for running.

Pass by the Botanical Garden's main entrance. You could drop in and see the gardens if you wish, but entrance to the gardens costs the astonishing fee of $12. This seems to me a strange but effective way of keeping the general public out. I feel sorry for the poor people who work hard building and maintaining what is undoubtedly a very pleasant and educational display, which is not then opened up to the people of Atlanta.

The path brings you out on Piedmont Avenue. Turn right and follow Piedmont northward a little way. After the end of the woods, there is a marked—but not light-controlled—pedestrian crossing across Piedmont Avenue. Take that crossing to the west side. Be careful— Atlanta drivers are not used to the concept of pedestrians trying to cross a road at a pedestrian crossing that does not have a stoplight.

A short distance north of the crossing there is an un-signposted street curving to the left into more peaceful territory—a residential precinct. You soon encounter a very pleasant suburban park, at the intersection of Avery Street and East Park Lane. Cut across the north end of this park and you come to the intersection of Maddox Drive and West Park Lane. Follow Maddox for about 50 yards across a creek and then turn left onto a foot path that follows the creek's west bank towards the southwest.

This is a very pleasant path, following a winding creek through Ansley Park, a zone of undisturbed native foliage, but never far from suburbia.

The path exits at Barksdale Drive. Turn left there. This takes you to the street called The Prado. Cross that street and do a dogleg towards the left, crossing the creek. Then continue following the creek on its left side to Lafayette Drive. You are here trekking adjacent to Winn Park, through a lovely suburban area. Turn right on Lafayette then left on Yonah Drive. Continue to 15th Street. Turn left on 15th Street to Piedmont Avenue. We found this route a very pleasant escape from Atlanta's typical urban environment.

Turn right on Piedmont and go one block south to 14th, by the main entrance to Piedmont Park. If you are ready for a food and drink break by now, there is an excellent establishment right here—the Prince of Wales pub.

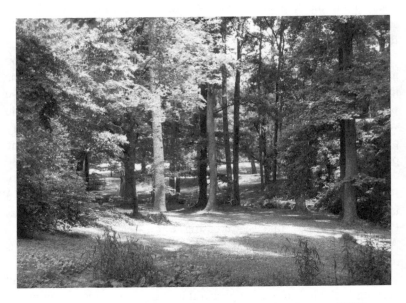

**Ansley Park—Beautiful Residential Parkland near Midtown**

This is very much a traditional English pub, complete with a red British telephone booth outside, but the food is better than that of many pubs in England. We found the company very engaging. This pub has been here since the early 1990s and has been such a success that it has recently spawned the start of a mini-chain of similar establishments in other parts of Atlanta. Should you not like the English pub formula, you can head west a couple of blocks to Peachtree Street where there are further restaurant choices.

To get back to the MARTA for transit to downtown, Buckhead, or other MARTA destinations, head west on 14th Street to Peachtree Street. Turn left and head south to 10th Street, then go two short blocks west to the MARTA station. Talk nicely to the token dispensing machine and, with luck, you'll get the token you need to whisk you wherever you want to go.

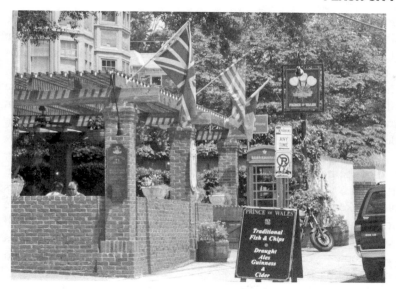

**The Prince of Wales—a Little Piece of England Hiding in the South**

# Other Ideas

**Grant Park**, in Atlanta's southeast quadrant, is recommended for running by some people, but locals always seemed to qualify that idea with "but be careful around there." I also read that it is in an area of "urban renewal," which usually is a euphemism for "slum undergoing redevelopment." We therefore decided not to consider it further. Maybe in a couple of years time, when the redevelopment is finished, this will be a great route. There is a large, historic cemetery close by, so it might make for an interesting destination.

An area that suggests itself as suitable for running is **Olympic/ Centennial Park** and its surrounds, site of the 1996 Summer Olympics. It is handy to downtown, in the southwest quadrant. However, we did not find a long enough runnable route for our criteria. Some people do run here, but it is a quite short loop and not outstanding. Major reconstruction projects in the area when we were there did not help with the pleasantness angle. Maybe it will be better some day in the future.

**Stone Mountain Park** is a winner in the attractions department but falls down on the convenience factor. It offers the sight of a huge granite monolith, with a 90-by-190 feet high relief carving of the likenesses of three Confederate heroes, plus a recreated 1870s town (called Crossroads), a museum, and various special events. It has excellent running conditions and scenery. Unfortunately, to get there, the only practical option is driving 16 miles on highways that are often congested. This place warrants a full-day outing by car, or even overnight camping, rather than being an urban on-foot route. However, definitely go there if you get the chance.

The **Silver Comet Trail** is a 37-mile trail constructed along the bed of the railway that carried the Silver Comet passenger train until 1969. It is a highly favored bicycle trail and also popular with runners and walkers. Like Stone Mountain, it falls down on the convenience criterion. To get to the trail's closest point to downtown, at Mavell Road SE, you need to drive. Furthermore, there is no way to build a circle route—you basically need to park your car at some spot then do an out-and-back course.

The **Chattahoochee River National Recreation Area** is a popular local recreation area outside the city in a northwesterly direction. It has several miles of runnable trails plus additional hiking trails. The only way I could find to get there is by driving, so we cannot really consider it an urban running destination.

Atlanta is well on the way to greatly expanding its urban system of bicycle and pedestrian trails. The **PATH Foundation** is dedicated to this cause. It has ambitious plans for 124 miles of trails overall. These plans include an 18-mile trail from Georgia Institute of Technology to Stone Mountain. We may have to wait a while before this project completes, but it will be an excellent asset when done.

* * * *

My bottom line on Atlanta is that there are definitely some great running trails outside the city, but generally they require automobile transport to get there. There are a couple of opportunities for interesting, enjoyable runs close to the city center and we have tried to pick out the best. As always, we welcome suggestions at our website.

Most importantly, we found the people of Atlanta to be just outstanding. Enjoy Atlanta! Now it is time for our tour to head to the Midwest…

# 7

# The Windy City

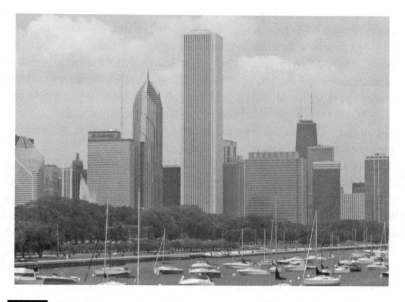

The Windy City is mighty pretty and a mighty pleasant place for on-foot exercise. Chicago, Illinois, is a city of history, culture, dedicated sports following, and more than a little charm. Its appeal for the on-foot exerciser is due, in particular, to the city's beautiful location on the western shore of Lake Michigan and to the city's diligence in making that entire lakeshore a parkland preserve.

Established in 1837, burnt to the ground in the Great Fire of 1871, and propelled to international recognition as host of the World's Columbian Exposition in 1893, Chicago has never been a boring place. Its most famous residents range from Abraham Lincoln, who was nominated for President in the 1860 Republican National Convention here (and subsequently elected to oversee the Civil War), to Al Capone, renowned mob boss of the 1920s.

There are plenty of things to do in Chicago. There are innumerable cultural, sporting, and entertainment events, and many excellent restaurants, pubs, and clubs. Winter tends to be somewhat chilly, keeping many people indoors, but in the rest of the year there is a strong outdoor culture. This includes on-foot activities. While runners and joggers mainly focus on a few favorite parks and trails, it is not unusual to encounter people jogging along city or suburban streets.

How good is the climate for outdoor on-foot activities? The three winter months of December, January, and February have average daily maximum temperatures around the freezing mark and a healthy snowfall, so don't plan on much on-foot activity other than winter sports those months. However, in the other nine months, the average daily maximum is in (or slightly above in July and August) our preferred 40-to-80 degree range. There is precipitation roughly one day in three year-round. This all adds up to pleasant running, jogging, or walking conditions from early spring right through late fall.

How safe is Chicago? The Capone-style gang warfare is a thing of the past. Chicago's violent crime index is 13.0[1] (crimes per 1,000 residents in 2003)—higher than average but significantly better than Washington and Atlanta. The locals will tell you that safety varies widely with locality. In general, people feel comfortable downtown and north of downtown, but areas south of downtown are more variable.

Chicago's road traffic is often a nightmare—especially the major arteries radiating from downtown to the more popular regional centers. However, the public transit system is very good. The Chicago Transit Authority (CTA) operates an extensive network of subways, elevated-line trains ("L"-trains), and buses. There are explanatory signs and maps posted at all stations and at many bus stops. There is an integrated fare system. The smart approach is to buy a stored-value Transit Card in advance for a few dollars. Transfers are cheap and computed automatically. The trains are fairly clean, and announcements are articulate.

The Blue Line subway to and from O'Hare Airport is a winner. It costs a couple of dollars between the airport and downtown and takes

---

1        Or possibly a little higher, since figures on forcible rape were not correctly reported to the FBI hence omitted.

45 minutes. When in Chicago on business trips, I sometimes took the Blue Line but often opted for the more business-like option of a cab or rental car. I can now tell you the truth: Every time I took the Blue Line I arrived on time and relaxed, whereas most times I was in a car (especially in peak hours) I was a nervous wreck and often late. I remember well those experiences sitting stationary in a vehicle on a jammed-up Interstate 90 watching the trains whiz by adjacent to the highway. Unless you have heavy bags or someone to impress, use the CTA for getting to or from O'Hare.

When it comes to selecting on-foot routes around Chicago, two routes stand out: the lakeshore north and the lakeshore south. We have run both of these several times and can indeed attest that they are both outstanding routes, satisfying all our criteria. The first of the two scores a little the better. We have also tried several other routes around Chicago, but everything else fell short. Therefore, we consider Chicago a two-route city.

| Route | Distance |
|---|---|
| 1. Lakeshore North—Navy Pier to Wrigleyville | 5.5-to-9.0 miles |
| 2. Lakeshore South—Navy Pier to Hyde Park | 7.9 miles |

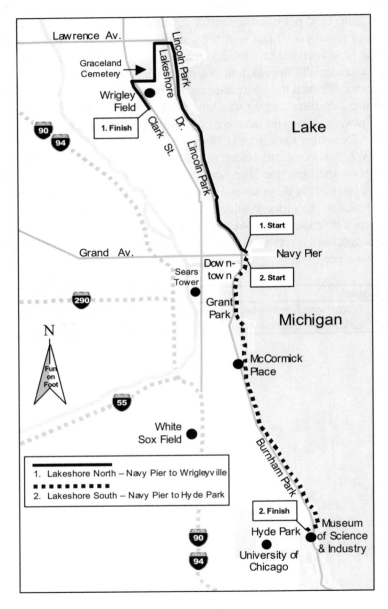

**Chicago Routes**

# Lakeshore North—Navy Pier to Wrigleyville

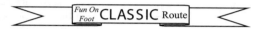

| Distance | 5.5-to-9.0 miles |
|---|---|
| Comfort | Most of the route is along flat, dedicated pedestrian or pedestrian/cyclist trails. The final one-to-two miles are along street sidewalks. Expect other pedestrians around, even on quiet weekdays. OK for inline skating. |
| Attractions | The natural beauty of the Lake Michigan shore, together with an attractive parkland setting most of the way. There are beaches, monuments, marinas, and sporting fields. After leaving the lakeshore, you enter a good quality mixed residential-commercial area. End near legendary Wrigley Field, home of the Cubs. In Wrigleyville there are many options for eating, drinking, and entertainment. |
| Convenience | Start at Navy Pier within short walking distance of downtown hotels. End in Wrigleyville, where there is fast and frequent subway service back downtown. |
| Destination | Some excellent bar/restaurants and a friendly local environment in Wrigleyville, the precinct of baseball's famous Wrigley Field. |

Our first Chicago route ranks highly in all our criteria. If you are in Chicago, and have even the slightest hankering for getting out on-foot and a couple of hours to fill, you must head north on the lakeshore.

Chicago's Lakefront Path runs roughly eight miles north and ten miles south of downtown. It has mile markers that give the distance from Bryn Mawr Avenue, its northern origin. Our suggested route here starts downtown and heads northward, but not quite as far as Bryn Mawr. We then head a short distance inland to the interesting wind-down destination of Wrigleyville.

We assume a start at Navy Pier—one of Chicago's main family-oriented tourist destinations. It is at the east end of Grand Avenue, off N Michigan Avenue, close to the city center.

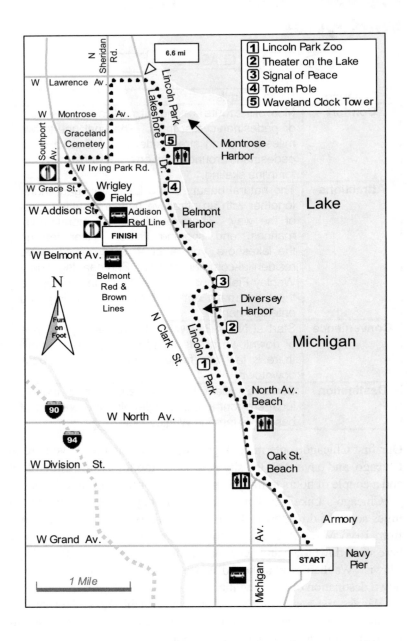

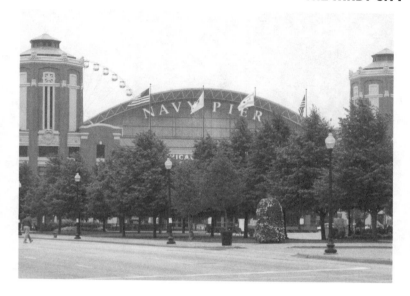

### Navy Pier

From the entrance to Navy Pier, follow the footpath northwest through Jane Addams Memorial Park to the lakeshore. You come to Ohio Street Beach, and link up with the Lakefront Path near its 7.5-mile marker.

The scenic Lakefront Path provides excellent running, jogging, and walking conditions. The track is wide. A big plus is an unsealed running path adjacent to the sealed bike path much of the way. We have sometimes met puddles on the unsealed path, but the sealed path is never far away. Water fountains are abundant on the Lakefront Path—so abundant we did not feel the need to note them on the map. Restrooms are also quite prolific. Chicago is truly exemplary in this respect. No other city makes water and restrooms so freely available on its urban trails. Winter, of course, is a different story—the water fountains and most of the restrooms will be disabled then, so be prepared.

With high-rises on your left and the sometimes-tumultuous, sometimes-placid lake waters on your right, the trail brings you to Oak Street Beach. Continue northward to W North Avenue. At this point Lincoln Park begins to take shape.

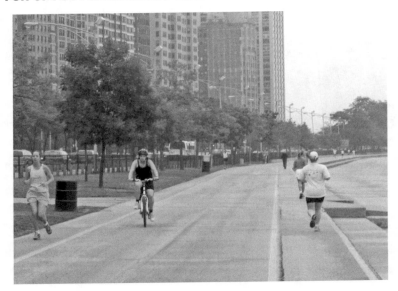

## Lakeshore Path North—Plenty of Room for All-Comers

Lincoln Park was established in honor of our 16th President shortly after his 1865 assassination. It has since grown to 1,208 acres, somewhat larger than New York's 840-acre Central Park. However, these two great on-foot venues are quite different in nature. Lincoln Park has the advantage of a lengthy attractive lakeshore. It also has the disadvantage of being draped around a major highway as its backbone, but that does not detract seriously from its appeal to the on-foot exerciser.

You arrive at North Avenue beach, where there is a kiosk and restrooms. From this point you can opt to either follow the beach or take the trail to the left through Lincoln Park proper. There is not much to choose between them—it depends on whether you prefer to see waves and sand or greenery.

If you take the inland trail, you pass on your left Lincoln Park Zoo. Established in 1868, it has a reputation as one of the nation's leading zoos, and one outstanding attribute—it is free. It is excellent to see a community opening up classy facilities to everyone this way.

If you take the beach trail, you pass Theater on the Lake. It has a café that is open evenings May through September. Cross the bridge over the entrance channel to Diversey Harbor. You then come to the

1890 statue of a mounted Indian chieftain, *Signal of Peace* by Cyrus Dallin, renowned sculptor of Indian figures and an ex-Bostonian. A little further on is another impressive statue—one of an Indian family with the inscription "To the Ottawa Nation of Indians—My Early Friends. Presented to Lincoln Park by Martin Ryerson." This was erected by the famed lumber magnate.

The two trails link up near the 3.5-mile marker (you have traveled a little over four miles from Navy Pier). Pass Belmont Harbor Marina on the right.

After W Addison Street, you come to the Totem Pole of Kwanusila, the thunderbird. You then pass a set of sports fields and, on the lake side of those, the fascinating ivy-cloaked Waveland Clock Tower and carillon, 1931.

---

**VARIATIONS**

You can cut our 9.0-mile route down to 5.5 miles by exiting the lakeshore at Addison. Take the pedestrian underpass under the highway to W Addison Street, and then follow W Addison Street to Wrigley Field and Wrigleyville. This preserves the end points and most of the main features of the route. Alternatively, to select an appropriate distance between the 5.5 and 9.0 mile options, you can leave the lakeshore at either W Irving Park Road or W Montrose Avenue, turn inland, and work your way south along the streets to Wrigleyville.

---

Our nominal route continues up the lakeshore to W Lawrence Avenue, with pleasant scenery all the way. Take Lawrence westward to N Sheridan Road, and then select your own route southward through the streets to W Addison Street and Wrigley Field. While you are now in ordinary streets, it is quite a pleasant neighborhood. We also passed a surprising number of runners on the streets, probably going to or from the lakefront.

Sheridan Road is quite pleasant to follow southward. Alternatively, if you go a further block west, you can go by Graceland Cemetery. There are many famous Chicagoans interred here, but it is not easily accessible to the public. While you can visit it via its Irving Park Road entrance, you cannot run (or even walk) through it from end to end.

Make your way to N Clark Street and W Addison Street. Here you find that famous ballpark—home of the Cubs, the "Friendly Confines"—

Wrigley Field. Built in 1914, Wrigley Field is the second-oldest major league ballpark, after Boston's Fenway Park, which opened in 1912.

As a Boston Red Sox fan, I have always felt certain empathy with the Cubs. The Cubs have not won a World Series since 1908 and not played in one since 1945. Their misfortunes since 1945 are blamed on the *Billy Goat Curse* laid by William Sianis during a 1945 World Series game, when the officials ejected his pet goat, Murphy, from Wrigley Field. This all sounds familiar to a Red Sox fan. Until the 2004 season, the Red Sox had not won a World Series since 1918 and this was blamed on the *Curse of the Bambino*, stemming from the trading of Babe Ruth to the Yankees in 1920. With the *Curse of the Bambino* broken in 2004, we all feel it is now time for the *Billy Goat Curse* to collapse too.

The area in the immediate vicinity of Wrigley Field has more bars and food joints than Sammy Sosa hit home runs in the 1998 season. So you will not go hungry or thirsty around here.

There are many places in Clark Street south of the field. We can recommend the Irish Oak, at 3511 N Clark Street. This Irish Pub is very popular with locals—every time we asked for recommendations it was suggested. The food and company were excellent. We have also eaten at John Barleycorn's at 3524 N Clark Street. It has a very attractive décor, including model tall sailing ships and 19th century paintings.

Another option is to venture a few short blocks west and north of Wrigley Field, to the area around the intersection of N Southport Avenue and W Grace Street. Here you escape from the hoopla of Clark Street and find some excellent eateries. At 4004 N Southport (at W Irving Park Road) is Deleece—our recommendation for the best Sunday brunch hereabouts, with traditional menu items as well as some more exotic choices. On Southport nearer to Grace there are more establishments, including our selection for Chicago's best Irish Pub—Cullens, at 3741 N Southport. This place has everything you could ever want in an all-round establishment—great food, a good selection of ales, friendly service, and ambiance.

Regardless of where, if anywhere, you decide to take a break around here, you will be close to fast public transit back downtown. Go to the Addison station, adjacent to Wrigley Field or, if you have drifted further south on Clark, the Belmont station. From either you can take the Red Line downtown.

---

# Lakeshore South—Navy Pier to Hyde Park

| Distance | 7.9 miles |
|---|---|
| Comfort | Almost all the route is along flat, dedicated pedestrian or pedestrian/cyclist trails. Expect other pedestrian traffic around, even on quiet weekdays. |
| Attractions | The natural beauty of the Lake Michigan shore, with a variety of scenery and sights along the way. Pass Grant Park, Soldier Field, McCormick Place, and Burnham Park. End near Jackson Park and the Museum of Science and Industry. OK for inline skating. |
| Convenience | Start at Navy Pier or elsewhere on the downtown lakeshore, within short walking distance of downtown hotels. End at Hyde Park where there is frequent bus (Route 6 or 2) or bus-subway (Route 55 or X55 to the Red Line) service back downtown. Catch the bus at the museum or at 55th and Hyde Park Blvd. |
| Destination | The Jackson Park/Hyde Park vicinity, with the Museum of Science and Industry and the University of Chicago nearby. There is an excellent all-round restaurant/bar at the end of the route, and several smaller ethnic restaurants. |

While the Lakeshore North route is our favorite, the Lakeshore South route comes a close second. There are fewer good food choices at the destination, and the public transit back downtown is not as convenient. However, the attractions are right up there—see Grant Park, the city's central playground, Burnham Park, site of the "Century of Progress" International Exposition of 1933-34, Jackson Park, site of the Columbian Exhibition that changed Chicago's face to the world in 1893, and the acclaimed Museum of Science and Industry.

Again we shall assume a start at Navy Pier. (If you staying in a downtown hotel pick up the lakeshore at the point most convenient to you.) From the entrance to Navy Pier, find the marked trail and follow it up to the street and then cross the Chicago River via the sidewalk of the road bridge. You are close to busy vehicle traffic here, but not for long—on the rest of the route you are generally well away from traffic.

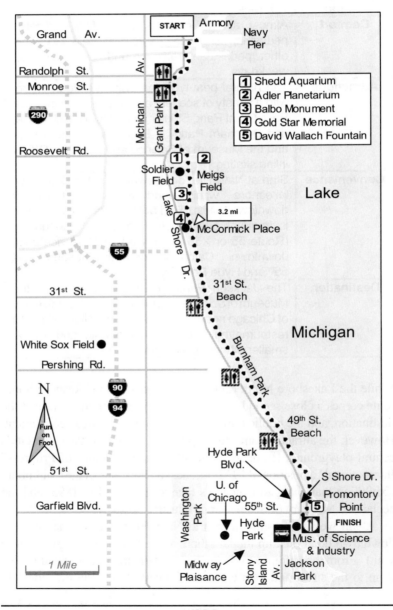

After the bridge, a couple of paths branch out—a pedestrian path immediately on the lakeshore and a marked bike trail. You may find large numbers of pedestrians and cyclists here, but the paths are wide so you should not feel crowded.

Enter Grant Park, the popular park area adjacent to downtown. There are plenty of facilities here, including restrooms and refreshment kiosks on the trail at E Randolph Street and at E Monroe Street.

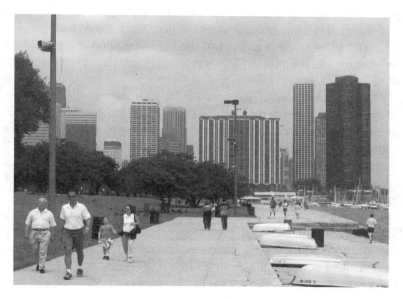

**Lakeshore South Pedestrian Path**

Continue to the trail's 9.5-mile marker, where you see the John G. Shedd Aquarium off to the left. The main path takes you around the back of the aquarium. Keep to the trail and resist the urge to go further out into the lake towards the Adler Planetarium and Astronomy Museum. There is no exit in that direction, since it is a peninsula accommodating the now-defunct Merrill C. Meigs airfield.

After the aquarium, the trail takes you around the lake side of Soldier Field, home of the Chicago Bears. The stadium originally opened in 1924. A massive reconstruction in 2002-3 amazingly produced a new modern stadium within the architectural shell of the original.

After Soldier Field, you come to one of the most amazing sights—a genuine, roughly 2,000-year old Roman column, standing on a fading pedestal—at the side of the trail. It proclaims itself as the Balbo Monument.

According to the inscription on its pedestal and the Chicago Historical Society[2], this column was a 1934 gift to Chicago from the Mussolini government. In that pre-war period, Mussolini was apparently trying to strengthen ties with the United States. For the past 60-odd years it has presumably been something of an embarrassment, since it is not generally promoted as a tourist attraction. What you may find most interesting about this strange artifact is that it still stands today where it was unveiled in 1934 in front of the Italian pavilion at the 1933-34 International Exposition. In fact, it is the only remaining standing relic of that famous event.

A little further on, at Waldron Drive, you come to the Gold Star Memorial, dedicated to members of the Chicago Police who gave their lives in performance of their duties. After that, you pass through the Chicago Fire Department Firefighter and Paramedic Memorial Park.

However, McCormick Place, Chicago's humungous convention center, soon dominates the space. The trail skirts this convention center on the lakeshore.

You can now settle down to some mindless, pleasant running, jogging, or walking along the scenic lakeshore. At E 31st Street, there is a swimming beach with restrooms, and shortly after the 13.5-mile marker there is a playground and more restrooms. At E 49th Street, there is another beach and restrooms. In warmer months you will find many local families enjoying these areas.

Around E 54th Street you come to Promontory Point. There is a very pleasant park here and, if you are still up for more on-foot action, it is worth a loop. However, if you keep to the main trail, you come to the David Wallach Fountain, decorated with a lovely bronze statue of a snoozing deer. Here is a good point to exit the lakeshore and start winding down. Take the underpass under the highway and bear left. You emerge at the intersection of S Shore Drive and E 55th Street.

On the left, you see Bar Louie. This is the best mid-market eating and drinking establishment in this part of town. Bar Louie has a comprehensive food menu (including its specialty, blackened catfish), a nice bar, a good crowd, and casual running gear is perfectly OK. Kids are welcome too. It opens at 11:00 daily.

---

2     Chicago Historical Society: http://www.chicagohs.org

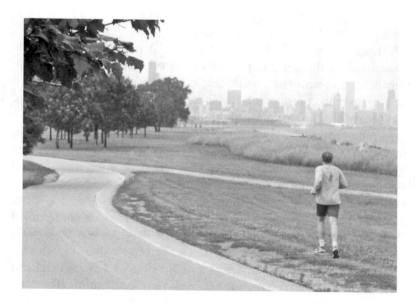

**Runners and Cyclists Use their own Paths**

The other big attraction around here is the Museum of Science and Industry. It is an enormous and impressive audience-participation-style science museum, and it is highly acclaimed. From Bar Louie, simply head two short blocks south.

To get public transit back downtown, catch a CTA bus either at the museum or at the intersection of E 55th Street and Hyde Park Boulevard (two short blocks west of Bar Louie). From either stop, you have two fundamental choices. You can take a direct bus to Michigan Avenue downtown or take a bus to the Red Line and connect to the subway downtown. We have tried both successfully and cannot recommend one over the other. The direct downtown buses are Routes 6 (Jackson Park Express) or 2 (Hyde Park Express in peak hours), which run express between E 47th and E 11th Streets. The buses to the Red Line are Routes 55 or X55 (Garfield). The latter buses will stop on the way at the Green Line, but we suggest you sit tight for a while and take the faster and nicer Red Line.

You have some other options to pursue while in this part of Chicago. You can take the opportunity to explore Jackson Park beyond the museum, the site of the 1893 Columbian Exposition. Alternatively, you have the opportunity to head west into the area known as Hyde Park, which houses the University of Chicago.

Heading west on E 55th Street (Hyde Park's main street) from Hyde Park Boulevard takes you past several small eateries. They include Japanese, Korean, Thai, and Middle Eastern restaurants, a bakery, and an up-market restaurant, La Petite Folie, at S Harper Avenue. The University of Chicago campus is southwest of Harper and 55th.

On the map of the Hyde Park vicinity, there are other green spaces that you might be tempted to explore on-foot. There is an impressive green corridor, called Midway Plaisance, located between E 59th and 60th Streets heading westward from Jackson Park. That is a great route to the University of Chicago, should you want to visit there, and it makes for a pleasant loop. There is also the green-space called Washington Park on the west side of Hyde Park. It is a large park, and was attractively designed and landscaped by—none other than... Frederick Law Olmsted, the designer of New York's Central Park, and various other places we have encountered in east-coast cities. However, I cannot enthusiastically recommend Washington Park for casual on-foot exercise today, since it is somewhat neglected and a little close to some not-so-desirable areas. You can certainly find better places to run in Chicago.

For public transit from Hyde Park to downtown, we suggest you catch the Route 55 or X55 (Garfield) bus anywhere in 55th Street to the Red Line. Unless you are really organized, don't consider the Metra train, which is fast but infrequent.

# Other Ideas

Chicago has its own "Emerald Necklace," also known as **The Boulevards**. This is a route of over 20 miles that links various major parks via streets with more than the average green space adjacent. While this is a fine concept, we had no success in trying to build a route that meets our criteria. There are two many traffic encounters, some questionable areas, and a lack of good destinations with convenient return transit.

The multi-mile **India Boundary Trail** follows the bank of the Des Plaines River on the western edge of Chicago. You can reach it via the Blue Line at Cumberland, almost at O'Hare. It does not meet our criteria but, if you like a little wilderness, it might be for you.

In case you thought that the Miracle Mile sounds like a nice place for a one-mile jog, we would caution you. For people interested in shopping-on-foot it is probably a winner, but that is it!

There are some other suggestions for running routes outside central Chicago in the *Chicago Running Guide*.[3] If you are a serious runner and spend a lot of time in Chicago, you will also find road race details in that book.

\* \* \* \*

To many people, the best-known part of Chicago is the terminal at O'Hare Airport, one of the nation's main airline transit hubs. Certainly I feel I know O'Hare at least as well as any other airport, even though I have never actually lived in Chicago. O'Hare does one little thing to brighten up your deadly dull layover—the bartenders ask *everyone* for an ID, just like at rock concerts or sporting events. People's reactions are interesting to watch. Younger people don't notice. More senior people, Americans at least, smile widely and are pleasantly surprised. The occasional person, usually a foreigner, is affronted—some even argue with the bartender. Oh, well; it is better than no entertainment at all…

On that little note, let us close our chapter on Chicago. Be sure to get downtown and experience the beautiful Chicago lakeshore on foot, every chance you get!

---

3       Brenda Barrera and Eliot Wineberg, *Chicago Running Guide*, Human Kinetics, 2000.

# 8

# Indy

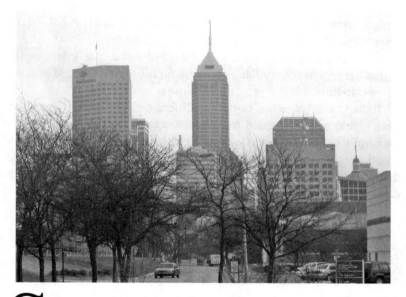

S tart your aerobic engines! We're off to Indianapolis, Indiana. Most people know this place for its signature role in the motor speedway game. While that role might reign supreme, Indianapolis has several other qualities that are less well recognized. From our personal experience, Indy is one of the nicest, most laid-back, and walker/jogger/runner-friendly cities in the country.

The establishment of Indianapolis was a pretty neat process. The Indiana State Legislature decided in 1820 to establish a brand new state capital in a sparsely populated wilderness area and to name it, quite simply, Indiana-polis (hyphen added by me for explanatory purposes). A nice tidy city plan was drawn up, the land was sold, and the city grew rapidly from nothing. The organized plan is still very evident today, with the entire city radiating in four quadrants from a center point—Monument Circle—with a straightforward street grid. Even the coming of the railroads later in the 19th century and the highway systems in the 20th century were planned quite sensibly and did not do enormous damage to the city's design.

Indiana's streets are very quiet, orderly, and clean. The vehicle traffic is generally quite light and drivers are relaxed. People are very friendly. The vast majority of people we passed on trails exchanged greetings with us. In fact, I would even go out on a limb and declare Indianapolis the most laid-back city we have covered in this book. The violent crime index (crimes per 1,000 residents in 2003) is 8.8—quite respectable, comparatively, for a U.S. city.

Another attractive attribute from the on-foot exerciser's perspective is that the region is very flat—there are no hills anywhere. If you are adverse to hills, this is a great place to run or walk!

Indianapolis' weather is not so different from Boston's or New York's, and generally good for outdoor activities. The average daily maximum temperature is in our preferred 40-to-80 degree range for six months of the year, with the other months just marginally falling outside that range one way or the other. There is precipitation on average 126 days of the year.

The public transit system, which comprises only buses, is not the best in the world. The buses are clean and people are friendly, but you really need to know in advance exactly where you are going and when. It is always a good idea to get a timetable in advance—the only bus needed for the routes described in this chapter is the No. 17 (College) bus, so you might wish to pull that timetable from the http://www.indygo.net/ website when you get a chance.

When it comes to selecting suitable on-foot routes in Indianapolis, that task has been simplified through the efforts of the Indy Parks and Recreation Department and the Indy Greenways Foundation. There is an extensive plan for pedestrian and bicycle trails, and implementation of this plan is well advanced.

My only negative comment is a paucity of water and restrooms on the Greenways trails. As with a few other cities, this deficiency really surprises me. Indianapolis' greenway planners have done an excellent job on most things but fall down badly in this department. Anyone designing greenway trails should be compelled to talk to Chicago's park and trail designers—they have shown how restrooms and water fountains never need to be a concern to park or trail users.

We have selected two routes for our coverage in this chapter, both of which satisfy all of our route-selection criteria very well. We think you will really enjoy these!

| Route | Distance |
|---|---|
| 1.  White River and Central Canal | 10.0 miles |
| 2.  Monon Trail | 7.1 miles |

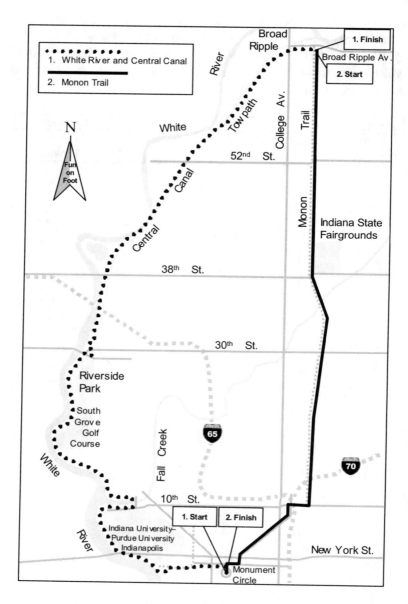

**Indianapolis Routes**

# White River and Central Canal

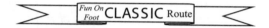

| Distance | 10.0 miles |
|---|---|
| Comfort | Almost the entire route is along flat, dedicated pedestrian/cyclist trails. Some of the route is adjacent to roads but much of it is remote from automobiles. Expect other pedestrians around, even on quiet weekdays. The second half of the route is not suitable for inline skating. |
| Attractions | The natural beauty of the White River and the Central Canal, generally devoid of automobile annoyances. Pass some notable places, including the downtown Canalwalk, Indiana University-Purdue University Indianapolis, the Indianapolis Museum of Art, and Butler University. |
| Convenience | Start within short walking distance of all downtown hotels. End in Broad Ripple, convenient to a bus service back downtown. Try to obtain a No. 17 (College) bus timetable in advance. |
| Destination | Some excellent bar/restaurants and a pleasant local environment in Broad Ripple. |

Our first route combines two Greenways trails—the White River Wapahani Trail and the Central Canal Towpath. This is an exceptionally good 10-mile route, with pleasant scenery, completely flat, on dedicated pedestrian/cyclist trails with cyclists in the minority. Trails are part paved and part gravel.

If you think 10 miles might be too far, take heart from Nola's and my story. When we were in Indianapolis researching this chapter, it was shortly after I had shoulder surgery. I had an arm in a sling, so running was out. However, we did not let that stop us—we just walked the entire route. We never had a moment of regret for that decision. We had an excellent half-day out on-foot, and really enjoyed that wind-down pub at the end! This is the type of quality route that you should not miss—regardless of whether you run, walk, or crawl.

Just one caution: Be sure to carry your own water, and don't expect much in the way of restrooms—there is only one on the route.

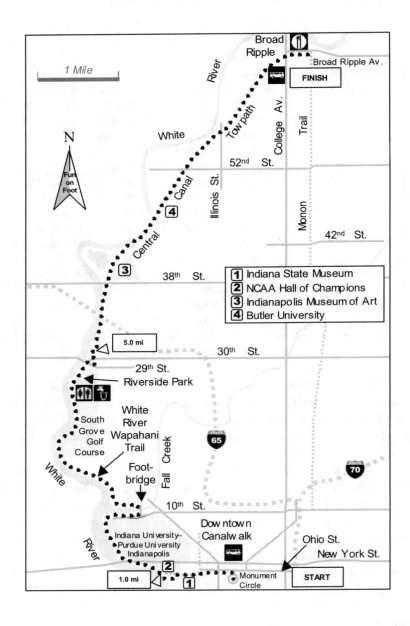

1 Mile

River

White

Broad
Ripple

Broad Ripple Av.

**FINISH**

Towpath

College Av.

Trail

N

Fun
on
Foot

52nd St.

Illinois St.

Canal

Monon

4

Central

42nd St.

3

38th St.

| | |
|---|---|
| 1 | Indiana State Museum |
| 2 | NCAA Hall of Champions |
| 3 | Indianapolis Museum of Art |
| 4 | Butler University |

5.0 mi

30th St.

29th St.
Riverside Park

White
River
Wapahani
Trail

South
Grove
Golf
Course

Fall Creek

65

Foot-
bridge

70

White

River

10th St.

Downtown
Canalwalk

Ohio St.
New York St.

Indiana University–
Purdue University
Indianapolis

2

1.0 mi

1

Monument
Circle

**START**

We assume a start in downtown Indianapolis, nominally at Monument Circle, the city's geographical center. However, you can easily find your way to the first part of our route from any downtown hotel or address.

Make your way to the downtown Canalwalk, running north-south roughly four short blocks west of the city's center. This piece of canal, and also the canal towpath we follow later in the route, formed part of the Wabash and Erie canal system intended to connect Lake Erie with the Wabash River, giving freight access ultimately to the Mississippi. The canals were built and operated in the mid-1850s but, as with most of the other canals of that time, were quickly obsoleted with the arrival of the railroad. The Canalwalk is very pleasant. It is a storey below street level with paved paths both sides and no cross traffic to concern pedestrians.

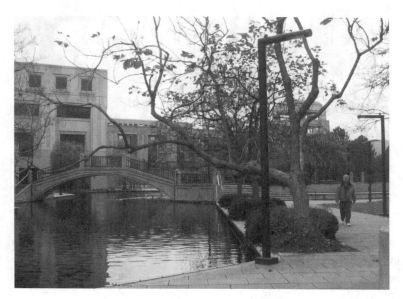

**The Downtown Canalwalk**

Follow the Canalwalk south to where it turns towards the west. Keep following the canal as it weaves past the Indiana State Museum, various state government buildings, and finally the NCAA Hall of Champions. At this point, the canal peters out, but keep following the path a short distance westwards to the bank of the White River.

Here you join the White River Trail. Head upstream on this nice, paved trail, generally well away from automobile traffic. On your right, you pass the campus of the university with a name designed for the Guinness Book of Records: "Indiana University-Purdue University Indianapolis." I'll bet it was fun watching the politicking that led to the adoption of that name! Even its common acronym "IUPUI" is unpronounceable.

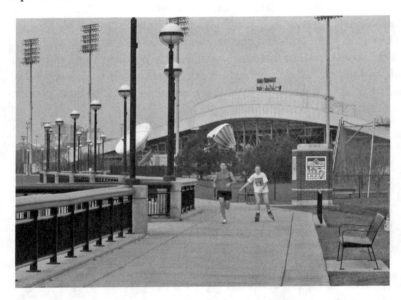

**The River Trail by the University**

At 10th Street the university campus ends and you come to the confluence of Rock Creek with the river. Follow the sidewalk around into 10th Street and proceed to the first light. Cross the road at the pedestrian crossing here. You shortly come to a footbridge across the creek, with an interesting, cable-stayed design.

After the bridge, follow the trail left back to the river. You pass a golf course on your right. According to some Indy Parks trail maps there is a public restroom at the golf course. I have no doubt there is one somewhere there, but don't be fooled. It is not convenient to the trail.

Continue past the golf course to Riverside Park. Here there really are restrooms, a water fountain, and a soda vending machine, although not right on the trail. You see in the middle of the park the Indianapolis

Recreation Center. Trek over to it if you are in need of any of those facilities.

In fact, this center even offers you the use of an excellently equipped gym for a token charge ($3 when we were there). If you have had too much of hotel exercise rooms, you have the opportunity for a nice weights workout in the middle of this on-foot outing.

Trek back to the river trail and continue upstream to 29th Street. You need to cross this busy street. Despite the traffic light, this crossing is still the most difficult part of the course.

After crossing 29th Street we suggest you leave the White River Trail (which you have already seen the best of) and pick up the Central Canal Towpath. First, you need to head east to bypass the Naval Armory. You then see signs directing you to the towpath. You need to turn left and circumnavigate a housing complex, but the trail is quite well marked. Eventually, after a few more signs, you come to the canal towpath. Go to the left (upstream).

At this point you have traveled five miles. You also have exactly five miles to go, along the towpath, to our suggested route end at Broad Ripple.

The towpath is gravel, flat, and well maintained. These are truly ideal on-foot exercise conditions (but not suitable for inline skating). The scenery is generally trees, greenery, and a watercourse—with residences not far away. In the first half of the trail, there is no vehicular traffic to be seen.

Ducks are prolific and brighten up the scene. They seem particularly happy ducks. There is no open season here.

We were on this trail in late fall, after most of the leaves were down. However, it was very obvious that this would be an amazingly beautiful place in the prime of fall. Don't miss that opportunity if you are ever presented with it!

After passing 38th Street, you are treated to views of a sequence of tastefully presented institutions across the canal. The first is the Indianapolis Museum of Art, which is attractively landscaped from the canal perspective. After that, you pass the Christian Theological Seminary, then the campus of Butler University.

The pleasant conditions continue up to the intersection with Illinois Street. Here, you need to cross the canal and follow the eastern bank. Conditions now change, for both the worse and the better. On the positive side, you will find some commercial establishments so, should you be badly in need of water or a restroom, you can at least buy a soda and beg an establishment for use of their restroom. On the negative side, you are now re-engaged with the automobile. The canal path from here on tracks a road with substantial—but not really heavy—traffic. Also, you are now faced with some trafficked roads to cross, but always with the assistance of traffic lights.

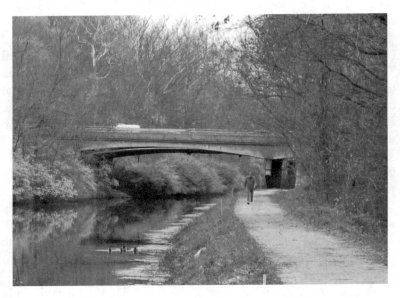

**The Central Canal Towpath is Pleasant all the Way**

Continue to College Avenue. Here you enter the Broad Ripple area. This is an attractive and lively place, an ideal destination for an on-foot route. There are many restaurants to choose from, including Mexican, Italian, Indian, Thai, Chinese, Sushi, and Applebees. There are also some excellent pubs.

We became attached to the Union Jack, on Broad Ripple Avenue two blocks east of College. It is one of the classiest English pubs outside England. It has been meticulously decorated, right down to stained glass windows, extensive artwork, and loads of English artifacts. The food was excellent, as were the staff. (The nachos were amazing!)

We also spent some time in the Broad Ripple Tavern, on Broad Ripple Avenue a block east of College. It is a more ordinary pub but had excellent food and company. There is also the Broad Ripple Brew Pub, which has good food but its drink choices are limited to beer brews—this may not work for everyone.

You can catch a bus directly back to downtown. However, get a bus timetable in advance—this is important! When we were there, the No. 17 (College) bus ran roughly half-hourly but every second bus took a slightly different route through Broad Ripple. Make sure you are waiting at the right place on the right half-hour —you would probably feel very unhappy sitting at a deserted bus stop for up to an hour, so do your homework on this. Another heads-up: Carry a few quarters and singles to pay the correct fare.

---

**VARIATIONS**

You can do this route in reverse if you want to end downtown. Alternatively, if you are prepared to go 17 miles, link this route with our following route.

---

# Monon Trail

| Distance | 7.1 miles |
|---|---|
| Comfort | Most of the route is along a flat, dedicated pedestrian/cyclist trail, with minimal automobile cross-traffic. Expect other pedestrian and cyclist traffic around, even on quiet weekdays. OK for inline skating. |
| Attractions | A peaceful absence of automobile traffic while following a high quality direct trail between two interesting end points—Broad Ripple and downtown Indianapolis. |
| Convenience | Start in Broad Ripple, reachable by the No. 17 (College) bus service from downtown. End within short walking distance of all downtown hotels. Alternatively, do this route in the opposite direction. If you are serious, you can link this route onto our first route to give a 17-mile loop from downtown. If using the bus, try to obtain a timetable in advance. |
| Destination | Some excellent bars and restaurants on your entry to downtown. |

This route has the same end-points as our prior route but is about three miles shorter. While still a quality trail, it is not as attractive as the first route. We assume starting at Broad Ripple and ending downtown; or if you want to go 17 miles in training for your marathon, tack this route onto our first route.

Despite claims on the Indy Parks Greenways map that there are several restrooms on the Monon Trail, we found this to be quite untrue—in late fall, at least. In early November, when on-foot conditions were otherwise excellent, there were no restrooms or water supplies at all on the trail. Perhaps they bring out some portable restrooms in the summer.

You find the Monon Trail crossing Broad Ripple Avenue roughly three blocks east of College Avenue. If traveling to the start of this route via the No. 17 (College) bus, ask the driver to drop you at the Monon Trail. Depending on which bus you are on, you will be dropped either on Broad Ripple Avenue or a half-mile south on Kessler Boulevard. Follow the trail southbound.

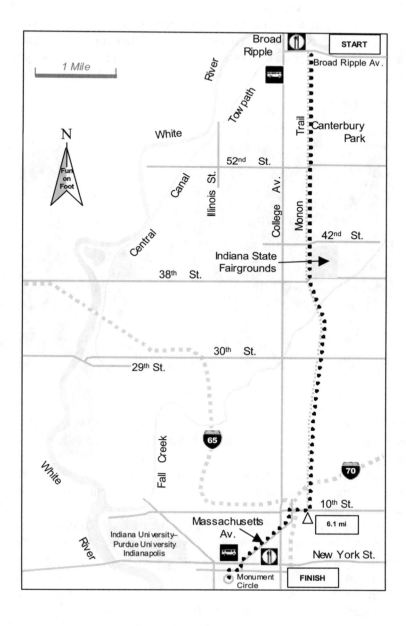

The Monon Trail uses the bed of the now-defunct Monon Railroad. It is fully paved, with gravel edges designed for pedestrian use. It is excellent for running. There are a few street crossings, but the drivers are generally very friendly and many give way voluntarily to pedestrians at these crossing points. There are helpful signs all the way, so you know exactly where you are.

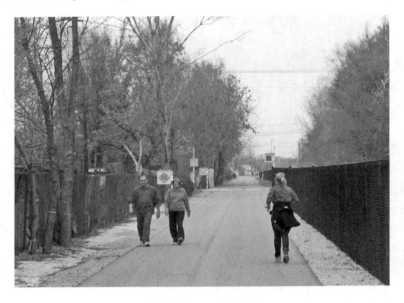

**The Monon Trail**

From Broad Ripple down to 54th Street the scenery is very attractive, with lots of trees and other plant life. You then pass the Indiana State Fairgrounds.

After the fairgrounds, the attractiveness declines. The trail is, after all, a rail trail, and the scenery you get is what you would expect along a suburban railroad track.

The trail ends at 10th Street, near the Interstate-65/70 interchange. To get to central downtown from here, you need to use street sidewalks, but the sidewalks are good and the streets are not particularly busy. Head westward on 10th Street and take advantage of its underpass under the freeways. Then turn left and pick up Massachusetts Avenue, the city's northeast-southwest divider. This street will take you directly to the center.

On Massachusetts Avenue you pass various eating and drinking establishments. Of particular note is the Rathskeller, Indy's oldest restaurant, established in 1894. It is in the historic Athenaeum building, at Michigan Street and Massachusetts Avenue. If you want something a little less ostentatious but with high quality food, drink, and fun, go on to MacNiven's Restaurant and Bar at New York Street and Massachusetts. This is a classy Scottish pub—one of a few of its kind in the United States.

You are now close to the city's center, and can easily navigate to Monument Circle or your hotel. There are many excellent restaurants and pubs close to the center, generally a little south of Monument Circle. For the aficionado of Irish Pubs, the place to go is the Claddagh Irish Pub on Meridian Street at Jackson Place.

# Other Ideas

Indy's greenway system has some interesting routes beyond those outlined above, plus extensive plans for the future.

The **Pleasant Run Trail**, following the Pleasant Run watercourse, extends from Ellenberger Park to Garfield Park south and east of the city. While we have no doubt this is a very pleasant run and is much enjoyed by locals, for travelers it falls down on the convenience factor.

The **Monon Trail** continues northward from Broad Ripple three miles to the county boundary and beyond. However, by this point, you are effectively outside the Indianapolis urban region.

What is more interesting is the set of future plans. The **Fall Creek Trail**, when completed, will connect the White River Trail to the Monon Trail, with an extension further northeast up Fall Creek. This will open up some attractive loop routes close to central Indianapolis. Several other trails are planned, and we eagerly look forward to completion of this roadmap.

\* \* \* \*

Indianapolis is not just the motor speedway capital of the United States—it is a very pleasant and relaxing place to visit, and offers excellent on-foot exercise and exploration opportunities. It has some dedicated greenway planners and some excellent on-foot trails that satisfy our criteria admirably.

Enjoy your time on-foot in Indy!

# 9

# Twin Cities

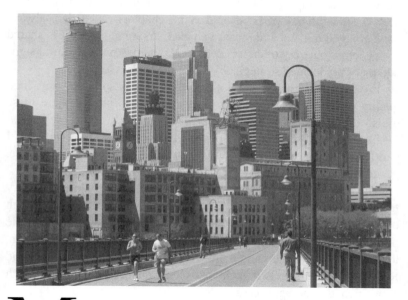

Minneapolis, Minnesota, is an abysmally cold and snowy place. In the winter, that is. However, from when the snow melts until the demise of the last Indian summer, Minneapolis is an amazing place for the on-foot enthusiast. The city has a very well developed urban trail system that caters for on-footers, as well as cyclists, in fine style. *Men's Fitness* magazine awarded this city honors for "Most Athletic City" plus "City That Watches the Least TV" for 2005.

While we titled this chapter *Twin Cities*, we must unashamedly admit that our entire coverage here is of Minneapolis—not its joined-at-the-hip twin, Saint Paul. This is not only because Minneapolis is the larger twin and attracts the more visitors, but also because the Minneapolis on-foot routes are just so outstanding they absorbed all our attention.

The biggest contributing feature to Minneapolis' trail system is the Grand Rounds—a 50-mile National Scenic Byway that weaves its way through and around central Minneapolis. It follows such scenic tracts as the Mississippi River, Minnehaha Creek, Chain of Lakes, and some of the other lakes that grace the urban area. The Grand Rounds is designed to serve motorists, cyclists, and pedestrians, in a way whereby none seriously impedes the other. In the most interesting and attractive sectors (including all parts covered in this chapter), pedestrians always have a paved trail separate from vehicles. In some places it is shared with cyclists but very often it is dedicated to pedestrians. Helpful signs and maps are located strategically along the trails.

In addition to the Grand Rounds, the city has some lengthy, high quality, commuter greenways. Cyclists and pedestrians share these trails, which generally follow old railway track beds.

Looking at the combination of these trails plus the city's substantial parklands, there are many attractive routes for on-foot exercise, generally a nice distance away from automobiles.

The public transit system is quite good; further making life easy for the pedestrian. There is a brand spanking new Light Rail through downtown and continuing south along Hiawatha Avenue. Its route includes such useful destinations as the airport and Mall of America, the nation's largest shopping mall. The Light Rail intersects the Grand Rounds at Minnehaha Park, helping us build quality on-foot routes with convenient downtown access.

The bus network is better than average. When boarding a bus or the Light Rail, you get a transfer good anywhere in the system for 2 ½ hours. Few outlets sell multi-ride tickets, so be prepared to carry a few singles and quarters for exact change. A stored value card, handy for the visitor to town, can be purchased at major transit centers. It works on any bus anytime but, unfortunately, does not work on the Light Rail unless you have transferred from a bus. Apart from that silliness, the system is straightforward and easy to use. We found all railcars and buses spotless and the staff very friendly and helpful.

For moving around central downtown, pedestrians have another big bonus—the Skyway system. This is a network of pedestrian paths weaving through the second floors of buildings, with glassed-in bridges linking adjacent blocks. While an excellent idea in winter, the system is something of a maze. Therefore, in good weather, you are probably better off simply using the street sidewalks. The street system is itself somewhat confusing. There is a numbered street and avenue system (think Manhattan, New York) but there are many weird angles and variations to the grid to confuse the unwary.

The average maximum temperature is in our preferred 40-to-80 degrees Fahrenheit range in April through November (actually it squeaks into the low 80's in July and August). However, in December, January, and February, the figures go down to the 20s. The community celebrates its non-winter months by strongly embracing outdoor activities, including running, jogging, and walking throughout the excellent trail system. Therefore, expect plenty of company while out on foot in this city. There is precipitation roughly one day out of three throughout the year.

The violent crime index is 11.9 (crimes per 1,000 residents in 2003), about average for all cities we cover. In the areas covered in our routes we saw no signs indicating particular problems. The routes generally traverse respectable residential areas, retail areas, or tidy parks, and the presence of other exercising pedestrians and cyclists is always reassuring. (As always, though, we cannot promise safety. You should take the usual precautions for any large city.)

There are various ways to slice and dice the Grand Rounds and the commuter greenways into nice 4-to-10 mile routes. We have put together five routes that meet all our usual criteria.

| Route | Distance |
|---|---|
| 1. Mississippi West Bank | 7.8 miles |
| 2. Downtown-Uptown Loop | 3.7-to-6.1 miles |
| 3. Chain of Lakes | 3.6-to-10.4 miles |
| 4. Minnehaha Creek and Lake Nokomis | 6.5 miles |
| 5. Cedar and Wirth Lakes | 8.2 miles |

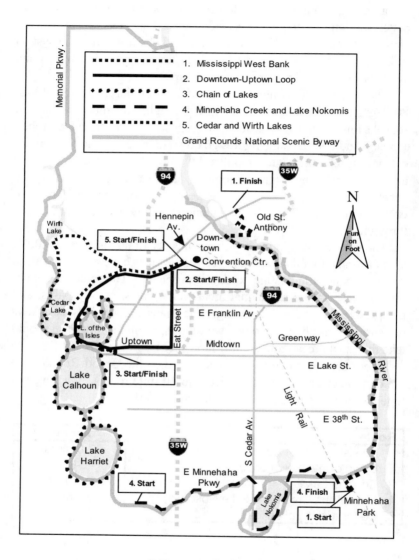

**Minneapolis Routes**

# Mississippi West Bank

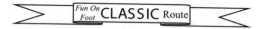

| Distance | 7.8 miles |
|---|---|
| Comfort | Excellent dedicated paved trails with no competing vehicle traffic, except for the last half-mile where ordinary street sidewalks are used. The trail is shared with cyclists in some parts. Expect other pedestrians and cyclists around but no crowds, except possibly for the last mile. OK for inline skating. |
| Attractions | Start in Minnehaha Park, with its own attractions such as the Minnehaha Falls. Follow a pleasant tree-lined parkway for the first part of the route. Follow the riverbank for the next part, passing Bohemian Flats and historic Mill Ruins Park. Cross the Stone Arch Bridge, follow the Saint Anthony Falls Heritage Trail, experience Old Saint Anthony, and explore the Central Riverfront District. |
| Convenience | Start at Minnehaha Park, easily reachable from all downtown points via the frequent Light Rail. End a short walk away from downtown hotels, shops, and the Convention Center. |
| Destination | Old Saint Anthony, the first settled part of the region. There are several historic sites and excellent wind-down eating and drinking establishments. |

This is our favorite route in Minneapolis, with high marks on all of the comfort, attractions, convenience, and destination criteria. The route starts at Minnehaha Park, south of downtown on the Mississippi bank, and follows the river upstream to the historic part of the city.

This route works equally well in the reverse direction—if you do that, see our fourth route description for more details of things you might want to see in Minnehaha Park afterwards.

Getting to Minnehaha Park is a breeze—just catch that pleasant and frequent Hiawatha Line Light Rail service anywhere on S 5th Street and take it to the 50th Street/Minnehaha Park station. After alighting from the railcar, cross the tracks and turn left along the pedestrian path past the preserved Princess Depot—a rail station from the turn of the century (19th-to-20th, that is).

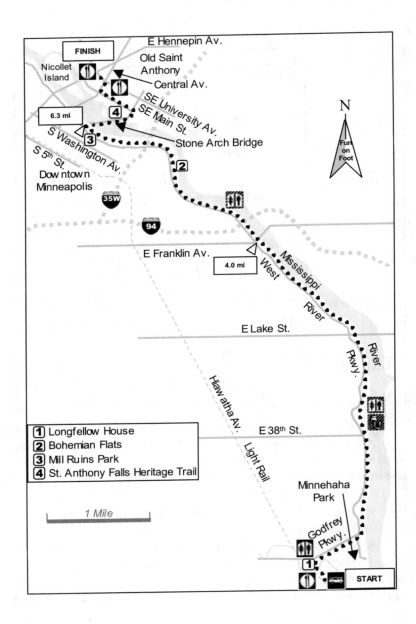

If you are new to the Minneapolis trail system, one worthwhile stop you can make here is at Longfellow House, where you find the Hospitality Center for the Minneapolis Park and Recreation Board and the Grand Rounds National Scenic Byway Interpretive Center. Here you can pick up a paper map of the Grand Rounds. The Longfellow House is a replica of Henry Wadsworth Longfellow's house in Cambridge, Massachusetts. To get to the Minneapolis Longfellow House, simply continue along the old rail track bed past the Princess Depot.

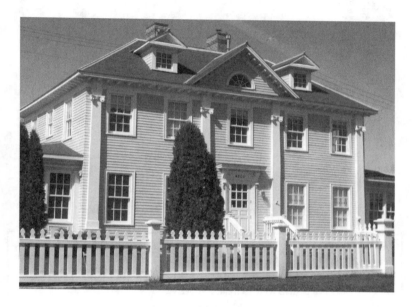

**Longfellow House**

Longfellow is a popular person in these parts; having immortalized the natural environment around here in his epic poem *The Song of Hiawatha*, completed in November 1855.

To get started on your route, follow the paved path to the northeast along Godfrey Parkway and then join the trail northward along West River Parkway. For the first part of the route, you are inland from the riverbank and cannot actually see the river. Nevertheless, the conditions are very pleasant. There are seasonal portable restrooms at a couple of locations. In addition to the occasional water fountain, Minneapolis has the interesting concept of hand pumps that serve up potable well water. We found these a little unreliable—sometimes you could get a good drink from one but other times it proved impossible to coax out even a drop.

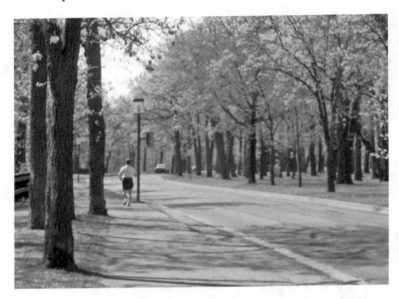

**Spacious Tree-Lined West River Parkway**

---

**VARIATION**

    Between E 24th Street and Minnehaha Park there is an alternative trail closer to the river—the historic Winchell Trail. There are various access paths to this trail. However, it is a dirt trail that is steep in parts and not always in the best of shape.

---

North of the Interstate-94 overpass the paved trail joins the riverbank. Pass the river flats known as Bohemian Flats. In the late 19th and early 20th centuries this was a developed area, with over 100 houses. Now it is a recreational strip, picnic area, and boat dock.

Continue to Mill Ruins Park and the Stone Arch Bridge. Mill Ruins Park is a historic site featuring the ruins of 19th century flourmills. This was the hub of the city's West Side Milling District (then the region's major industry) and the largest water powered facility in the world. Excavations have revealed mill footings, canals, and other parts of the waterpower system serving the mills.

Cross the Stone Arch Bridge, once a rail bridge but now the province of pedestrians and cyclists. From the bridge you can see the ongoing Mill Ruins excavations, the Saint Anthony Falls (the only waterfall on the Mississippi), and the modern-day lock and dam system. The first hydroelectric station in the United States began supplying power at St. Anthony Falls in 1882.

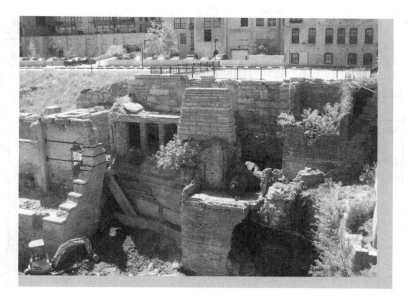

**The Mill Ruins as Seen from the Stone Arch Bridge**

After crossing the bridge you are in Old Saint Anthony, where settlement of the region commenced in 1848. Head upstream into Father Hennepin Bluffs Park, adjacent to Main Street. This area forms part of the Saint Anthony Falls Heritage Trail—you may find the trail's historical markers illuminating. In Main Street between the Stone Arch Bridge and Central Avenue, there are also several eating/drinking establishments with outdoor patios. This is a pleasant place to wind down from your on-foot exercise.

If you head north one block to SE University Avenue then turn left, you come to another interesting part of Old Saint Anthony. At the intersection with Central Avenue you find Ard Godfrey's house, the oldest remaining house in the City of Minneapolis, built in 1849.

Godfrey was a millwright, postmaster, and miller from the region's earliest days.

There are several other eating and drinking places around here. We particularly liked Keegan's Irish Pub, on NE University Avenue just past E Hennepin Avenue. It has great food and an immaculate, rich, wooden interior shipped from Ireland. We spent a long time talking to the publican and bar staff, and learnt a lot about the area.

To get back to downtown from here, the simplest way is to walk across the Hennepin Avenue suspension bridge straight into the center of downtown. However, you may well want to take the opportunity to explore other parts of the Central Riverfront District, including Nicollet Island and Boom Island Park, while here.

---

**VARIATIONS**

If you want to extend this route southward, the trail continues beyond Minnehaha Park to historic Fort Snelling. There is also a Light Rail stop there.

Alternatively, if you want to extend this route northward a little, you can continue up the river on the Saint Anthony side, through Boom Island Park, then cross the river back to downtown at 8th Avenue NE (North Plymouth Avenue).

---

# Downtown-Uptown Loop

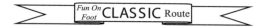

| Distance | 3.7-to-6.1 miles |
|---|---|
| Comfort | Dedicated paved trails or good street sidewalks with little vehicle traffic the first 4.8 miles. Regular street sidewalks are used the last 1.4 miles. The trail is shared with cyclists in some parts. Expect other pedestrians and cyclists along the entire route. Crowds are unlikely to be a problem, except possibly for the first mile. Not recommended for inline skating (except the lakeside trail). |
| Attractions | Loring Park, the city's central park, the Sculpture Garden with its impressive outdoor creations, a classy residential neighborhood, and the scenic edge of one of the city's most attractive lakes, Lake of the Isles. For the final section, traverse Eat Street, a 17-block stretch of ethnic restaurants; either eat here or pick out a place to come back to in the evening. |
| Convenience | Start and finish in the heart of downtown on Nicollet Mall, handy to the Minneapolis Convention Center and most downtown hotels. You can optionally cut the route short at 3.7 miles, ending in Uptown where you can catch a bus back downtown. |
| Destination | Nicollet Mall in downtown Minneapolis, with its excellent restaurants, bars, and shops. You also have two other options. You can end in Uptown, where there are some good wind-down food-drink establishments, and frequent buses back downtown. Alternatively, if you would like a broad choice of ethnic restaurants at the end of your outing, stop in Eat Street, with its 17 blocks of restaurants. |

If you are staying or working in downtown Minneapolis and have limited time to get away on foot, this is a nice route to give you a taste of the Chain of Lakes and introduce some good eating and drinking destinations. You will also learn some of the key secrets of the Minneapolis on-foot trail system.

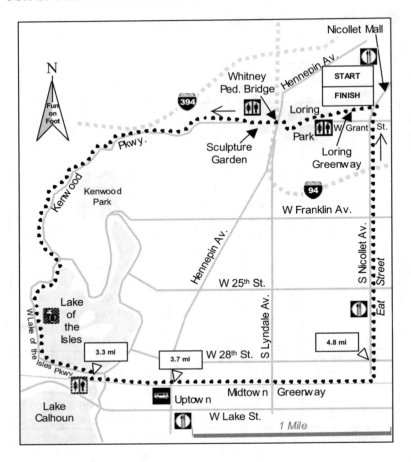

We start this route on the Nicollet Mall at S 12th Street, near the Hyatt Hotel and handy to the Minneapolis Convention Center. Here you find the not-so-obvious entrance to the Loring Greenway, a very handy pedestrian thoroughfare heading west to Loring Park.

Proceed through the Loring Greenway and enter Loring Park near the landmark Benjamin Berger Fountain. Loring Park is Minneapolis' closest equivalent to a central park, not very big, but scenic, close to the business district, and popular. It was named after Charles Loring, the first superintendent of the Minneapolis park system. Given the state of this outstanding park system today, he certainly deserves the recognition.

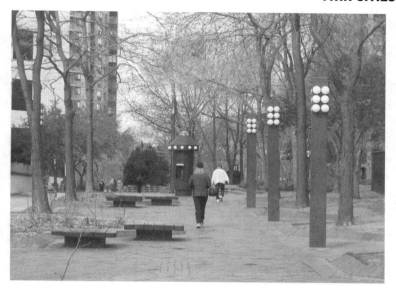

## Loring Greenway—Downtown's Secret Escape Route

Continue straight ahead through Loring Park, and navigate the Woodland Circle. This part of the park, started in 1998, will eventually be a woodland garden of native wildflowers, shaded by birch trees. Cross the quaint bridge over the creek and continue in the same direction to the Whitney Bridge—the blue truss-structured pedestrian overpass over Interstate 94 and Hennepin Avenue.

Cross the bridge and enter the Minneapolis Sculpture Garden, an 11-acre park that gives everyone an opportunity to see works of art by leading sculptors in a garden setting. There are restrooms inside the greenhouse complex. Entry is gratis.

Proceed straight through the Sculpture Garden and emerge on the north sidewalk of Kenwood Parkway. Follow the sidewalk past the parking lots. After a short distance, you pass a pedestrian/bicycle trailhead that takes you to the Cedar Lake Trail. Don't take that now—we'll discuss that option in our fifth route.

Kenwood Parkway is a pleasant, winding, tree-lined, residential street. Keep following it up and down a hill or two until you come to its end at West Lake of the Isles Parkway.

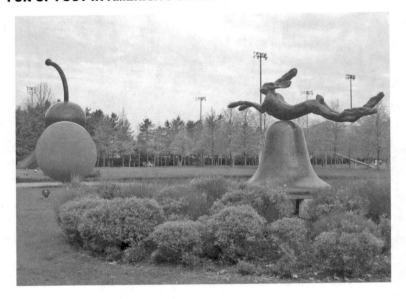

**Minneapolis Sculpture Garden**

Minneapolis has several lakes. However, they don't get much better than Lake of the Isles. It is beautiful, peaceful, and has magnificent homes the length of the parkway. There is a paved trail around the lake, usually dedicated to pedestrians. Cyclists have one big disadvantage here—they are restricted to going clockwise around this and the other lakes in the Chain of Lakes. It is good to be on foot and have the freedom to choose which way to go.

We suggest going counterclockwise around this lake. In due course you reach the lake's south end and the road heading further south to Lake Calhoun. You have some choices here. For now, we suggest you simply climb the trail connector to the Midtown Greenway (also known as the 29th Street Greenway).

---

**VARIATION**

To add 3.1 miles to this route you can head south here, do a loop of Lake Calhoun, and pick up the route again here. See our next route description for more information on Lake Calhoun.

---

The Midtown Greenway is a valuable asset for the on-footer in Minneapolis. It uses an old rail track bed, generally following 29th Street across the city. The trail is shared with cyclists but there are separate lanes for those folk. Take the trail eastward.

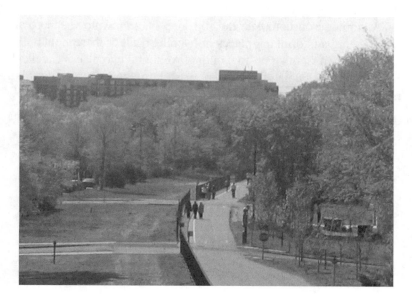

**The Midtown Greenway**

You are entering the Uptown area. If 3.7 miles is far enough for you, it makes sense to get off the Greenway at Hennepin Avenue. You can get a bus back downtown from right here if you wish. However, Uptown is an interesting place in its own right, so you might wish to follow Hennepin a block south to W Lake Street where there are shops, restaurants, bars, and action.

The best restaurant around here for an on-foot wind-down is Figlio, at the intersection of Hennepin and Lake. This is a popular place with a big sidewalk eating area, ideal for a nice sunny day. There is a good selection of foods, slanted towards the Italian but plenty of choice overall. Brunch is offered on Sundays.

To continue with the full route, go a further mile along the Midtown Greenway from Hennepin Street and exit at Nicollet Street. Follow Nicollet Street to the left, heading north. It is about 1.4 miles along the Nicollet Street sidewalk to where this route started in Nicollet Mall.

What is particularly interesting about this part of Nicollet Street can be deduced from its moniker—*Eat Street*. This is the city's biggest, if not best, restaurant strip. There are restaurants of various cuisines stretching several blocks along this street, almost to downtown. If you decide to eat here, you can easily walk back downtown afterwards.

Assuming you complete the full loop back downtown, there are many eating and drinking places in Nicollet Mall or thereabouts. For winding down from an on-foot outing, we found two places excellent: Brit's (English) Pub and The Local (Irish Pub), both on Nicollet Mall near the Loring Greenway and both with sidewalk tables.

# Chain of Lakes

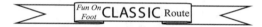

| Distance | 3.6-to-10.4 miles |
|---|---|
| Comfort | Excellent dedicated paved trails, except for the street sidewalk used on the last half-mile. The trail is shared with cyclists in some parts. Expect other pedestrians and cyclists around for the entire route. There may be quite a crowd on a nice summer day, but the trails are spacious enough to accommodate everyone. Vehicles will not impede you. OK for inline skating. |
| Attractions | One of the best 10-mile pedestrian trails you will find anywhere. There is attractive scenery throughout and outstanding conditions. |
| Convenience | Start and end in Uptown, roughly two miles south of central downtown. It is easily accessible by frequent No. 6 and No. 12 bus services in Hennepin Street. Alternatively, you can combine parts of this route with parts of our second route. |
| Destination | Uptown, where there is much activity, some good wind-down food-drink choices, and frequent fast buses back downtown. |

*Chain of Lakes* is probably the best-known catch-phrase for on-foot activity in Minneapolis. This city has lots of lakes and several of them are close enough to combine into nice on-foot routes. However, the heart of the Chain of Lakes is unquestionably the trio of: Lake of the Isles, Lake Calhoun, and Lake Harriet. Distances around the pedestrian trails of these lakes individually are 2.6 miles, 3.1 miles, and 2.75 miles, respectively.

We nominally start and finish in Uptown, at the intersection of Hennepin Avenue and W Lake Street. As explained in our first route, you can easily get to and from here by bus or on-foot and, if so inclined, you can add a mile and make Eat Street your destination.

Take the Midtown Greenway from Hennepin to where you see the water, and then follow the sidewalk a short distance north to Lake of the Isles. This description assumes you will circumnavigate all lakes counterclockwise, but you can choose to go the other way or go different ways on different lakes if you prefer.

Go completely around Lake of the Isles to where you started. Then follow the road south, going under the Midtown Greenway. You come to Lake Calhoun, the largest of the lakes.

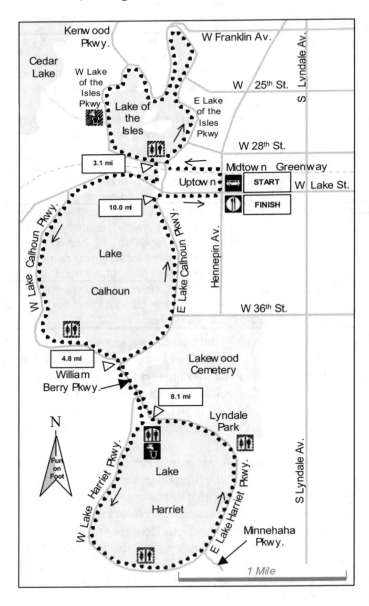

---

**VARIATION**
   If 3.6 miles is your limit, call it quits here and head back to
Uptown on the Midtown Greenway.

---

Bear right and go around Lake Calhoun to the main road at its
southern end, William Berry Parkway. Follow William Berry Parkway
to the north end of Lake Harriet.

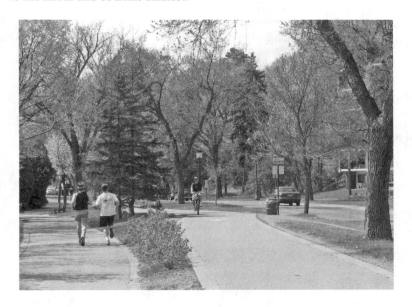

**Separated Pedestrian, Bike, and Car Trails Around Lake
Calhoun**

---

**VARIATION**
   If 10.4 miles is too far for you, skip Lake Harriet and continue
around Lake Calhoun. This brings the total distance down to 6.5
miles.

---

As you approach Lake Harriet, you see a very attractive pavilion
ahead, with characteristic tall round roofs. There is an entertainment
area here, a café that is open seasonally on limited days, and real
restrooms (not the smelly portable variety). Head to the pavilion then
proceed around the lake counterclockwise.

---

Lake Harriet is as pretty as the others, with winding treed trails and many beautiful homes along the parkway.

After getting back to William Berry Parkway, follow its sidewalk back to Lake Calhoun. Then follow the Lake Calhoun east-side trail north to W Lake Street, and take that street east to Hennepin Avenue where you started this route.

Have a wind-down snack and drink at Figlio and catch a bus in Hennepin back to downtown.

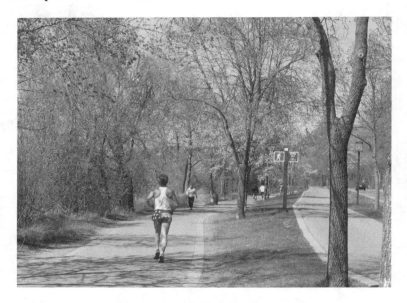

**The Trail on Lake Harriet East**

# Minnehaha Creek and Lake Nokomis

| Distance | 6.5 miles |
|---|---|
| Comfort | Dedicated pedestrian or pedestrian/bicycle trails all the way with plenty of shade.  Expect other people around the entire route, but no crowds.  Very relaxing route.  OK for inline skating along the bicycle trails, but not in Minnehaha Park. |
| Attractions | A particularly attractive route from the nature perspective, with much greenery, a babbling creek, and a lake with wide grassy surrounds.  End at Minnehaha Park with its scenic and historic attractions. |
| Convenience | Start at S Lyndale Avenue and W 50th Street, easily reached via the No. 4 bus from downtown.  End at Minnehaha Park with convenient transit back downtown via the frequent Light Rail. |
| Destination | Minnehaha Park with its attractive and famous falls, and historic sites including John H. Stevens House and the Princess Depot. There is great down-home style food at Cap's Grill. |

This route covers the south leg of the Grand Rounds: Minnehaha Creek; a loop of Lake Nokomis; and a finish in Minnehaha Park, with its various attractions and convenient Light Rail service back downtown.  This is the route that Nola and I agreed is the most beautiful on the Minneapolis menu from the natural environment perspective. You follow wide, treed parklands all the way.  There are always people around, but crowds are unlikely.  There is a dedicated pedestrian path almost the entire way.

The route starts at S Lyndale Avenue and W Minnehaha Parkway. Assuming you are coming from downtown, take the No. 4 bus in Hennepin Avenue to S Bryant Avenue and W 50th Street.  We found the bus service frequent enough on weekdays but it can stretch to 30 minutes on Sundays.  On alighting, head south on Bryant to the parkway then two short blocks east to S Lyndale Avenue.

At our start point, the bike trail is effectively the parkway's south sidewalk so start off just following that eastward.  In due course it will lead you down and closer to the creek and a separate pedestrian trail spins off.  This is a very pleasant trail, with plenty of greenery and shade.

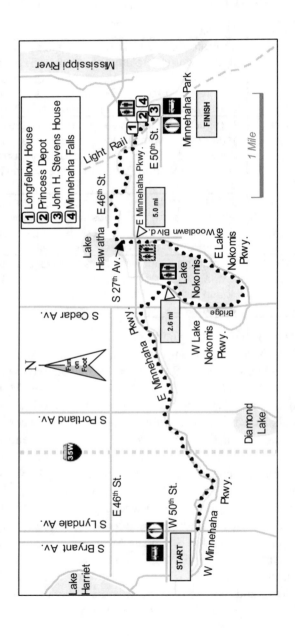

**VARIATION**
    You can tack this route onto a half-loop of the Chain of Lakes, giving a total distance of roughly 14 miles. To do this, take the W Minnehaha Parkway from the southeast corner of Lake Harriet (see our previous route) to our nominal start point of this route.

Continue to the bridge at S Cedar Avenue. Follow the trail under the road then loop back onto the bridge and cross it to the south side. Angle across the sporting fields to the left. This brings you to the northwest corner of Lake Nokomis. There is a beach here and a refectory with restrooms and, on limited days in season, a snack bar.

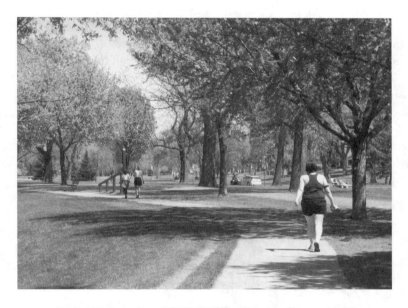

**Lake Nokomis with Its Wide Grassy Surrounds**

Lake Nokomis (originally Lake Amelia) received its new name in 1910 to honor Nokomis, grandmother of Hiawatha. It is a very pleasant lake, with a wide grassed area and excellent paved trails around it. Start going around the lake counterclockwise. When you reach S Cedar Avenue, you have a choice of either continuing on the lakeshore or taking a shortcut along the sidewalk of the S Cedar Avenue bridge.

Continue around the lake to its northeast corner, where there is a park access road to E 50th Street and Woodlawn Boulevard. Follow Woodlawn Boulevard north to E Minnehaha Parkway, cross that road, and continue north on S 27th Avenue to Minnehaha Creek and the south end of Lake Hiawatha. Lake Hiawatha is dominated by a golf course so is not of much interest to us on-footers.

Pick up the paved trail eastward along Minnehaha Creek. It is very pleasant here, since you are removed from the parkway and its vehicle traffic. Continue to where you can see the Light Rail tracks and meet up again with the parkway. Take the bridge over the tracks to arrive near Longfellow House (discussed in our first route).

You now have an opportunity to explore Minnehaha Park, and its attractive and famous Minnehaha Falls. It also contains several historic sites including the John H. Stevens House (1850), the first wood frame dwelling built west of the Mississippi, and the Princess Depot, a restored railway station from the 1900s, now housing a small museum.

To get back to downtown or other transit destinations, go south a short way to E 50th St. and the Light Rail Station.

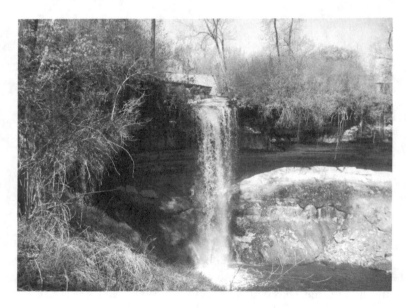

**Minnehaha Falls**

If you feel like some food, we have one great recommendation, Cap's Grill. It is just across Hiawatha Avenue from the Light Rail station. It is a very friendly, down-home style establishment boasting the Twin Cities' best barbequed pork ribs, best pork chops, and best weekend breakfast. There is brunch on Saturdays and Sundays. The place is closed on Mondays. No alcohol is served.

---

**VARIATION**

You can do this route in the opposite direction, although there is not much to see or do when you arrive at S Lyndale Avenue. There is a nice little restaurant in W 50th Street near Bryant, and you can conveniently catch a bus back downtown from there.

---

# Cedar and Wirth Lakes

| Distance | 8.2 miles |
|---|---|
| Comfort | There are paved dedicated pedestrian or pedestrian/bicycle trails most of the way, with a few sections through parks or on street sidewalks. Expect other people around most of the time, but fewer than on our other Chain of Lakes routes. Crowds are unlikely except for the park sections near the start and finish. Parts of the route are not suitable for inline skating. |
| Attractions | Good escape from the bustle and the cars of the city, passing two lakes not included on prior routes. Pass through Loring Park, the Sculpture Garden, and (optionally) the Eloise Butler Wildflower Garden and Bird Sanctuary. |
| Convenience | Start and finish in the heart of downtown on Nicollet Mall, handy to the Minneapolis Convention Center and most downtown hotels. |
| Destination | Nicollet Mall in downtown Minneapolis, with its excellent restaurants, bars, and shops. |

Our final route would be classed outstanding in any other city. However, in Minneapolis, it is verging on the mediocre, since it is not as stunningly beautiful as other routes. However, it has the attribute of being a downtown-to-downtown loop on dedicated trails with amazingly few traffic encounters. It is ideal for a city hotel dweller or city worker with a couple of hours to spare and a desire to escape from the hordes and the traffic. Some of the ideas might also be mixed with elements of our second and third routes to tailor something special.

We start the same as in our second route, on Nicollet Mall, downtown near the Hyatt Hotel. Take the Loring Greenway to Loring Park, go straight through that park, and take the blue pedestrian bridge to the Sculpture Garden. Proceed straight through the Sculpture Garden and emerge on the north sidewalk of Kenwood Parkway.

Follow the sidewalk past the parking lots on your right. After a short distance, you come to a trail entrance on the right with a sign indicating the Cedar Lake Trail. Follow the path to Interstate 394, go under the highway, and then meet up with the trail proper.

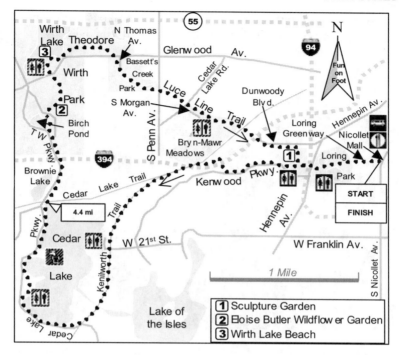

Sculpture Garden
Eloise Butler Wildflower Garden
Wirth Lake Beach

The Cedar Lake Trail is a very impressive development, connecting downtown with western communities. Like many other bicycle/ pedestrian trails, it follows the bed of a disused railway track. However, it is generously designed, with three separately paved paths—one for pedestrians and one for each direction of bicycle traffic.

Take the trail heading west. After less than a mile, the trail splits, as do the accompanying railroad tracks. The right-hand branch goes north of Cedar Lake and continues west. Take the left-hand branch, known as the Kenilworth Trail, which heads clockwise around Cedar Lake. Conditions continue to be excellent. You do not see the lake shore just yet. At W 21$^{st}$/22$^{nd}$ Street, you can divert west across the rail tracks to a small park on the lakeshore; there is a portable toilet there.

Keep on the main trail to Cedar Lake Parkway. Turn right following the Grand Rounds pedestrian trail from here. Follow the trail around the south edge then west edge of Cedar Lake. This trail is not as popular as some of the other lake trails in Minneapolis, which you might consider a plus or a minus. Underfoot conditions and the general surrounds are very pleasant, but don't expect crowds. The lake is lovely and has various spots popular with bathers, kayakers, and fisherpersons.

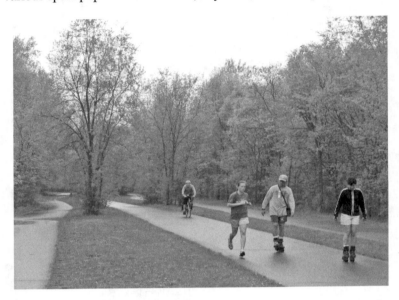

### The Kenilworth Trail Comfortably Accommodates Everyone

At the north end of Cedar Lake, there is a bridge over the rail track and the Cedar Lake Trail—that is, the trail going north of the lake, which we earlier chose not to follow. Cross the bridge via its sidewalk and continue following Cedar Lake Parkway northward.

Cross the bridge over the interstate and follow the pedestrian path along Theodore Wirth Parkway. You pass a vehicle exit road. Shortly after that the pedestrian trail heads off on its own, away from the Parkway and into Theodore Wirth Park. Follow that pedestrian trail until it intersects a one-way vehicle road.

At this point you face a decision. You are adjacent to the Eloise Butler Wildflower Garden and Bird Sanctuary. If you want to traverse that area, turn right and follow the pedestrian trail to its main gate. Then enter the garden and work through it to its back gate. The garden is an interesting place and entrance is free, but it is not ideal territory for the serious runner and out of the question for inline skaters. Your other choice is to keep following the main pedestrian trail straight ahead to the cross-trail intersection.

If you negotiated the wildflower garden, exit at the back gate and take the trail to the left, which leads to the same cross-trail intersection.

From the cross-trail intersection, follow the paved trail north a short distance to where it meets Glenwood Avenue. Cross Glenwood Avenue and follow the pedestrian/bicycle trail east to the facilities at Wirth Lake beach. When we were last here, there was considerable maintenance and reconstruction work going on, but after that is complete we expect this to be a very pleasant place to traverse or to sit down and take a break.

Follow the trail eastward, just north of Glenwood Avenue. We found the trail poorly marked for the next part, so take care. Cross the Glenwood Avenue bridge over the rail tracks and turn right into N Thomas Avenue. Push on, and after a while you find a marked trail starting up again. This is the Luce Line State Trail. It is quite a pleasant stretch, threading through parklands adjoining residential areas.

At one point the trail peters out and you need to take the street sidewalk south to cross two bridges over the railway tracks and the creek. Then take S Morgan Avenue to the left. This brings you into the Bryn-Mawr Meadows area, with extensive sporting fields accommodating such not-so-common sports as cricket. (I was somewhat surprised to see two serious cricket games under way the day I was here.)

Follow the paved trail through the sporting fields. It brings you to a big pedestrian overpass over what, to us, looked like a Mad Max demolition zone of old railway yards and industrial facilities. Obviously something good will happen here in due course. Regardless, the trail and the bridge are very sound, so it all works fine for the on-footer.

The bridge takes you to a point where you must choose to either take the city end of the Cedar Lake Trail to downtown, or bear right and take the street under the interstate to Dunwoody Boulevard. The latter, which we think is more pleasant for the pedestrian, takes you back to the northern edge of the Sculpture Garden. You can cross Dunwoody, enter the Sculpture Garden, and retrace your footsteps through Loring Park and the Loring Greenway to Nicollet Mall. You end handy to the Minneapolis Convention Center, major hotels, shops, and some excellent wind-down eating/drinking establishments.

# Other Ideas

If you look at our citywide trail map at the start of the chapter, you will see many possible ways of combining parts of our route recommendations to produce your own variants. I hope the information we have given will help you do that.

As to the Grand Rounds, we covered all but the most northern parts, which generally lack the outstanding qualities of other parts from the on-footer's perspective. However, one northern part of the Grand Rounds you might wish to visit is **Memorial Parkway**, with its rows of trees, markers, and memorials commemorating the Hennepin County servicemen of World War I, plus other notable folk. You can also take in the beauty of Shingle Creek and the North Mississippi Regional Park nearby.

We did not say much about the **Central Riverfront District**, which is possibly the most popular and interesting on-foot area in central Minneapolis. Since that area is more suited to wandering and exploring than to four-mile-plus exercising, we figured we would just leave that area to you.

The city also has several **commuter bike trails** beyond those we have mentioned. Some of these extend substantial distances into the suburbs. We hear they are great for serious running training, but they do not fit our urban on-foot recreational trail criteria so well.

* * * *

Why does the coldest, snowiest major city in the 48 states have the best trail system for non-winter on-foot exercise? I don't know for sure, but I suspect it is no coincidence. I see similar trends in other wintry cities, like Chicago, Boston, Denver, and the Canadian cities I have lived in. Maybe winter-burdened folk develop a special appreciation of the importance of outdoor fitness activities.

Regardless, anyone living in or visiting Minneapolis is blessed with an outstanding set of on-foot route choices to help build fitness and to enjoy. Make the most of it!

# 10

## Big 'D'

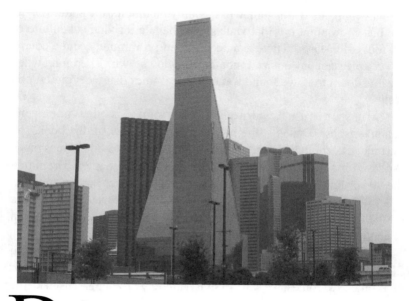

Dallas, Texas, is the world's largest shopping mall. It is such a big mall, in fact, that people have to drive their cars from shop to shop. Walking is, by and large, an alien concept here. If you asked the average person what was the most important thing he did with his feet, he would say hitting the accelerator and the brake.

The Dallas road system is, to say the least, highly developed. But there is one really quaint thing about Dallas streets—the romantic street names. For example, there are "Lover's Lane," "Mockingbird Lane," and "Walnut Hill Lane." Takes you right back to the rural English countryside, no? The problem is that these cutely named streets turn out to be major, multi-lane highways—so much for the quaintness and the romance.

As a pedestrian, life is not always easy. Dallas people are the friendliest you will find anywhere, but the cars are the least friendly. Obviously a Texan undergoes some kind of transformation upon getting behind the wheel. Streets often have sidewalks, but one gets the impression they were designed by someone who has never used a sidewalk. A Dallas sidewalk is typically a five-foot concrete strip immediately abutting eight or more lanes of fast-moving traffic. Nola remarked how the cars zoomed by so close that she feared someone in a car might snatch her bag as it went by!

Having painted that somewhat gloomy picture for the pedestrian let me hasten to point out that Dallas does have a thriving subculture of on-foot enthusiasts. There is a keen running community, and a couple of very pleasant on-foot trails not far from downtown. Therefore, when it came down to it, we found some on-foot routes that meet our criteria well.

Let us start, as usual, with a quick look at some general environmental characteristics. Dallas is the hottest place we cover in this book. Its average maximum temperature is in our desired 40-to-80 degrees range for seven months, but exceeds that in May through September, hitting the 90s in June through August. Therefore, if you are here in summer, you might go to extra pains to fit your outdoor exercise in early in the day. The average number of rainy days per year is 79, so precipitation is relatively unlikely to cause you problems.

Dallas' violent crime index is 13.7 (crimes per 1,000 residents in 2003), higher than we like to see. However, in the areas around our recommended routes, we saw no signs of safety problems. Just take the usual precautions of any large city.

Dallas public transit, the DART bus and light rail system, is middle-of-the-road, with respect to its quality as well as where its rail tracks often run.

The two light rail services are modern and immaculately clean. However, they are not as frequent as one would expect and the stops seem a long way apart. (But, of course, Dallas is BIG.) The ticket machines are a disaster—the ticket purchase process is more a battle of wits between man and machine than a simple business transaction. One machine delayed me so much I missed my train.

When it came down to finding suitable on-foot routes, we were helped enormously by our friend Steve, a serious local runner. However, we also did some exploring cold. For example, we wandered downtown looking for the start of the Katy Trail (highly recommended by Steve and others). We bravely sauntered into the downtown Information Center and asked them. The people there were very friendly and helpful, like most Dallas folk. However, our question seemed to stump them. Four staff members worked on this question for quite some time, and eventually came up with not quite the right answer. It was clear that none of them had ever actually been on the Katy Trail.

We ended up putting together two excellent routes, which build upon three local on-footers' favorite places—the Katy Trail, Turtle Creek, and White Rock Lake. We mixed in a few twists and variations to satisfy our convenience and destination criteria. We hope you will enjoy these routes or devising your own routes from their ingredients.

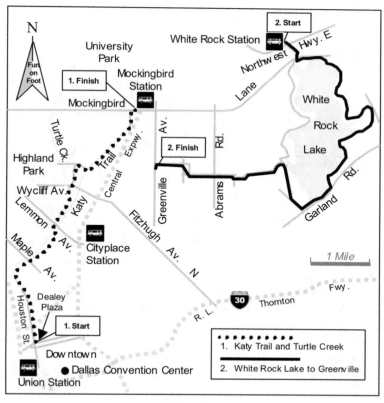

**Dallas Routes**

| Route | Distance |
|---|---|
| 1. Katy Trail and Turtle Creek | 5.2 miles |
| 2. White Rock Lake to Greenville | 9.1 miles |

# Katy Trail and Turtle Creek

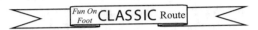

| Distance | 5.2 miles |
|---|---|
| Comfort | Almost all the route is along flat, dedicated pedestrian or pedestrian/cyclist trails. There are short stretches near the start and finish on street sidewalks. Expect other pedestrian traffic around, even on quiet weekdays. The Katy Trail is good for inline skating, but not Turtle Creek. |
| Attractions | Downtown sights, including Dealey Plaza and American Airlines Center; a pleasant dedicated pedestrian/cyclist trail; a suggested diversion to take in attractive Turtle Creek and some outstanding Highland Park mansions; and a finish at an excellent Irish pub near a busy shopping area and Southern Methodist University. |
| Convenience | Start downtown within short walking distance of the Dallas Convention Center and downtown hotels. End convenient to a DART Rail station at Mockingbird, with fast service back downtown. |
| Destination | An excellent Irish pub/restaurant, Trinity Hall, with shops and cinemas adjacent. Easy access to the Mockingbird DART station. |

The Katy Trail was built over the bed of the former Missouri-Kansas-Texas (MKT or *Katy*) Railroad. The railway, which began operation in 1887, was the main link between Dallas and the East Coast for many decades. After 100 years of operation, the Katy Railroad tracks were abandoned.

The end result, thanks to the efforts of the Friends of the Katy Trail organization,[1] is one of the finest examples of "rail trail" development

---

1      The Friends' website is: http://www.katytraildallas.org

in the country.　It provides pedestrian/cyclist access through a major community corridor, with important end-points—Downtown and Mockingbird. Furthermore, it is a rail trail that has succeeded admirably in shaking off the urban railroad track imagery, such as industrial back doors, junkyards, and undesirable dwellings—a problem that other rail trails often face. On the contrary, the Katy Trail traverses an environment of lush greenery through high quality inner suburbs, and provides a very effective escape from automobile-based Dallas mainstream life.

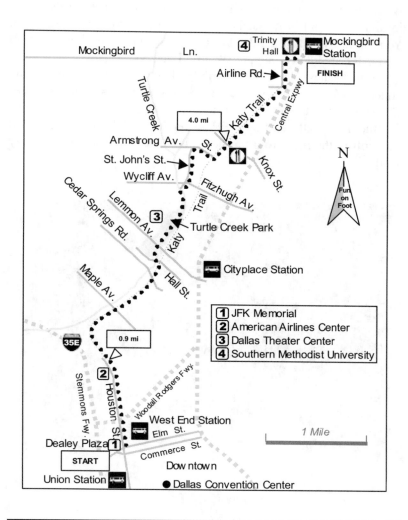

It so happens that near the Katy Trail, for part of its length, is Turtle Creek, an older, and more established parkland area. Turtle Creek is blessed with its own, unique watercourse-based beauty, and proximity to some impressive buildings. Therefore, we are presented with the exciting opportunity to build on-foot routes that can take advantage of both environments. This gives pedestrians an opportunity for much more variety than the typical cyclist!

The route starts in downtown Dallas. For our nominal start point, we have selected the most famous spot in Dallas—Dealey Plaza, the location of President Kennedy's assassination on November 22, 1963. You can easily walk to Dealey Plaza from any downtown hotel, or from the DART at Union Station or West End Station.

From Dealey Plaza, head north on Houston Street. After going under the Woodall Rodgers Freeway you come to the American Airlines Center, home of the (NHL) Stars and the (NBA) Mavericks. Continue past the arena on the east side of Houston Street. Take the foot trail that bears off to the right from the sidewalk. This is the start of the Katy Trail.

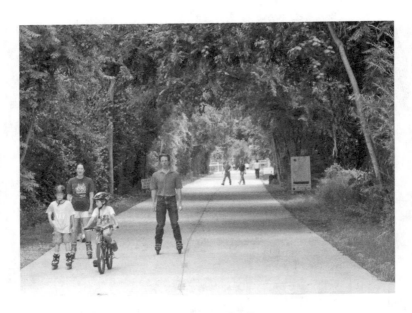

**The Katy Trail**

The Katy Trail is a 10-foot wide concrete trail, shared by pedestrians and cyclists. When we were last on it, there were more runners, walkers, and families with small children than there were cyclists. It was certainly very pleasant. It is planned to add an adjacent 6-foot wide, soft-surface track made from recycled running shoes. When done, this will make for a truly outstanding urban trail.

Turtle Creek runs alongside and west of the Katy Trail for roughly the first half of the Katy's length. This opens up an ideal opportunity for on-footers to divert from the Katy Trail for part of the route to experience some different scenery and conditions. I would suggest leaving the Katy Trail around Cedar Springs Road or Hall Street.

---

**VARIATION**

If you are on inline skates or are pressed for time, just stick on the Katy Trail. You will shorten the route a little that way, but miss out on some attractive scenery.

---

We chose Hall Street, where we could conveniently scramble down the old railway embankment to the street below. (Be careful of a possibly slippery slope, though!) Cross the creek at Hall, and then follow the Turtle Creek Trail northwards on the west side of the creek.

The Turtle Creek trail is unquestionably more attractive than the Katy Trail. You can expect more peace and quiet, and no bicycles at all. There is a flowing stream, and ducks, geese, and other wildlife abound.

Keep following the main trail northward. Cross Avondale Avenue, and then bear right away from Turtle Creek Boulevard. Cross Fitzhugh Avenue, and find St. John's Street. You are in the classy suburb of Highland Park. If you are not impressed by St. John's Street, with its green space on one side and stately mansions on the other side, then you do not impress easily. Continue to Armstrong Street, and turn right. The properties in Armstrong are also impressive. These streets present typical examples of the glorious up-market housing for which Dallas is famous.

Armstrong Street ends at the railway easement. Here you will find a convenient short footpath up to rejoin the Katy Trail. Turn left, taking the trail northward.

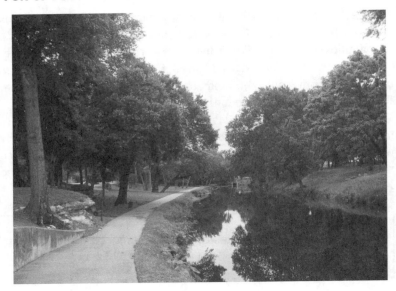

## The Natural Beauty of Turtle Creek

You soon come to Knox Street, which is a point where you might consider taking a break if you need one. There are several restaurants and pubs very close to here. Nola and I did this route on a very hot day and weakened to take an enjoyable drink break at the On the Border Mexican Grill and Cantina, on Knox very close to the trail.

Break or no break, continue up the Katy Trail to its end at Airline Road. When we were there, work was still in progress and it was not clear exactly how this trail termination would finish up. However, what worked best then, and will still likely work in the future, is to follow the Airline Road sidewalk north to Mockingbird Lane. Attractive Airline Road has several quite regal brick homes, generously decorated with gas-burning lamps. Busy Mockingbird Lane is a different story—follow its sidewalk eastwards across the mind-numbing Central Expressway and cross to the northern side.

You are now in our recommended destination area, handy to the DART Mockingbird Station. Proceed on Mockingbird to where you see the DART tracks disappearing underground, then head north into the shopping area.

If you are inclined towards a food or drink wind-down from your exercise, we have a great recommendation here. Trinity Hall, upstairs in the shopping area, is an exceptionally good Irish Pub. It has an interesting and pleasant décor, and serves excellent food from a widely varied menu.    Trinity Hall is modeled on Dublin's Trinity College, complete with a collection of differently styled seating areas, including the Provost's Corner, the Library, the Student Union and, of course, the bar.

An advantage of Trinity Hall, if you are on foot is that, when you exit, you walk right into Mockingbird Station with Red Line and Blue Line trains to take you back downtown.

Not many urban routes satisfy our formula as well as this one!

# White Rock Lake to Greenville

| Distance | 9.1 miles |
|---|---|
| Comfort | The first 6.5 miles are along flat, dedicated pedestrian or pedestrian/cyclist trails. The remainder is along quiet street sidewalks. Expect other pedestrian traffic around, even on quiet weekdays. OK for inline skating. |
| Attractions | A very attractive lakeshore route, well removed from the automobile world, with excellent quality trails and plenty of wildlife. We tack onto this a short route through an attractive residential suburb to reach a superior eating/drinking destination. |
| Convenience | Start at the White Creek DART Rail station and end at a place where you can either walk a mile to DART Rail, or catch a local bus there or downtown. |
| Destination | One of Dallas' best eating, drinking, and entertainment areas, especially popular with locals for weekend brunch. |

White Rock Lake is the most popular running, jogging, and walking place in Dallas. It is a sizeable, attractive lake, originally a reservoir, surrounded largely by parklands. There is a nine-mile trail around it, accommodating pedestrians and cyclists. It is a popular venue for racing events for both runners and cyclists.

The most common approach by locals is to drive here (you can park in lots off Mockingbird Lane or Garland Road) and run or walk a loop of the lake. If you have a vehicle, that is a fine approach. However, as usual, we looked for an option that does not require a vehicle and that has an interesting eating and drinking area as its destination. We found it possible to link up a White Rock Lake partial loop with a destination in what most locals would agree is the finest weekend brunch area in the city.

To start, take the Blue Line DART Rail to White Rock Station. At the traffic lights, cross Northwest Highway East. (Are you starting to get confused with Dallas Street names yet?) Also cross W Lawther Drive, where you find a trail heading south. Follow this pleasant trail down to Mockingbird Lane, which you can cross via a pedestrian underpass.

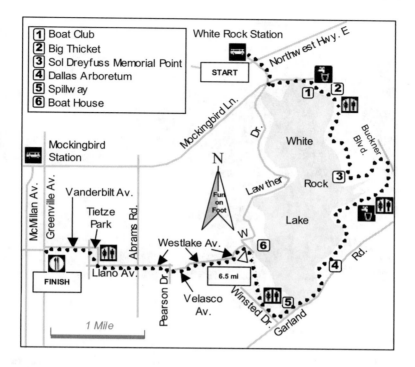

The better side of the lake is the eastern side—the paths are wide, automobiles are scarce, and you are treated to some excellent views of the western lakeshore and the downtown skyline in the background. Turn left after the Mockingbird underpass and take the bridge sidewalk across the creek. (There are some nice little local trails near the lakeshore here, but they will not lead you to the eastern lakeshore—you need to use that road bridge!)

After the bridge, follow the first road to the right. It takes you to the lake. You soon find some nice pedestrian-friendly dirt trails that bypass the road (which is closed to through traffic anyway).

This is a very pleasant area for on-foot exercise—excellent underfoot conditions and a beautiful environment. There are also restrooms and water fountains at various points. Pass the White Rock Boat Club and the Big Thicket. You come to a point jutting into the lake, called Sol Dreyfuss Memorial Point. Here you get an excellent scenic view westward.

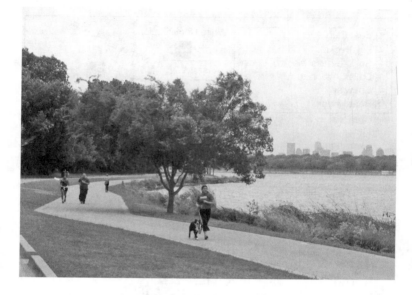

**White Rock Lake with City Skyline as Backdrop**

The trails then force you towards the east to negotiate two creeks which enter the lake. After crossing a bridge over the major creek, the path swings back westward. After getting back to the lakeshore, you pass the Dallas Arboretum, with Indian teepee and covered wagon nearby. You then come to the spillway—an interesting environmental area, with very impressive bird life.

You are forced onto the street sidewalk to negotiate the spillway. After the spillway, keep bearing right following Winsted Drive, and then pick up the main pedestrian and bicycle trail towards the northwest. Keep to the main paved trail, which is straight and follows an old railway bed.

At the end of the long straight stretch of trail you can see the Boat House area ahead and to the right. Take the natural trail spur to the left to W Lawther Drive and follow that street two short blocks to Westlake Avenue. You are now leaving the lake and moving into a classic, but particularly pleasant, suburban residential area.

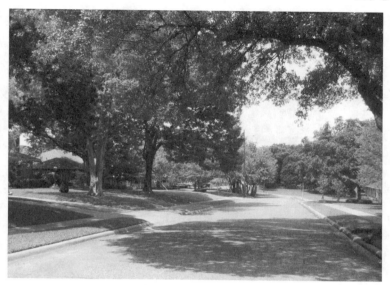

**Westlake Avenue**

---

**VARIATION**

If you drove to the lake or want to head straight back to the White Rock DART station, keep following the western lakeshore around to where you started, rather than leave the lake here. If you start and finish at the DART station, the total route length is 10 miles (or 9.1 miles if you park in one of the lakeshore parking areas).

---

Follow Westlake to where it becomes Velasco Avenue. Take Velasco to Pearson Drive, turn right, and then left back onto Westlake. Follow Westlake to Abrams Road, where it changes name to Llano Avenue. Continue to Tietze Park, where there are restrooms.

Head west on any of the streets here—Vanderbilt (at the north end of the park) is probably the nicest. Proceed to Greenville Avenue where, if you are in an eating or drinking mood, you will find a very welcome destination.

This is one of Dallas' best eating, drinking, and entertainment areas, especially popular for weekend brunch.

---

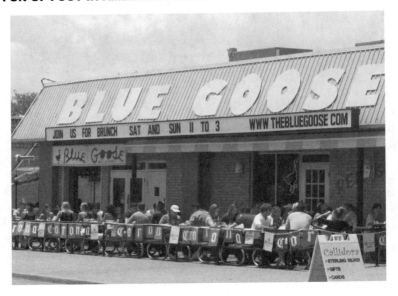

**The Blue Goose, a Typical Greenville Brunch Spot**

There are several restaurant and bar choices. The Blue Goose Cantina is a popular Mexican restaurant, with homemade tortillas. The Hurricane Grill is a New Orleans Oyster Bar, Terilli's is an Italian Restaurant, and the Greenville Bar and Grill is a good all-round place. All of these places serve Saturday and Sunday brunch. Other establishments include the Dubliner Irish Pub but you would not go there for the food.

Returning to downtown requires a little effort from here. Mockingbird DART Station is a little over a mile away, 14 blocks north and three blocks west. If you feel like some exercise to help the digestion, you should do this walk. Alternatively, go due west two blocks to McMillan Avenue and catch a local bus to either Mockingbird Station or directly downtown.

## Other Ideas

The 7.5-mile **White Rock Creek Trail** connects Valley View Park in North Dallas to the northern tip of White Rock Lake, where our second route starts. Valley View Park is just north of Interstate 635 at Hillcrest Road. The trail is cement paved and is popular with cyclists and inline skaters, but not so much with pedestrians. Locals say the White Rock Lake loop is much more comfortable and attractive. Furthermore, Valley View Park, while being a convenient place to park, is not convenient to public transit.

**Bachman Lake**, northwest of downtown just beyond Love Field, has a paved 3.3-mile trail around it. The park is popular with families and with local runners for 5K runs, but is sometimes crowded. Furthermore, there is little to do nearby and some locals cautioned us about the safety of the surrounding vicinity.

When one looks at the map of Dallas, what stands out from the green space perspective is the significant length and massive width of the Trinity River and its banks. Why, asked I, are there not a set of beautiful parks and running trails through there? The answer, I was told, is that the city is still reserving the right to dredge the river and open a major port here.

However, this reservation does not extend upstream to the Elm Fork Trinity River and the West Fork Trinity River, which feed the Trinity River proper. Dallas' westerly municipal neighbor, the City of Irving, has put in place a program to build a major trail system right through here. Known as the **Campion Trails**, there is already a short trail section on the Elm Fork and another on the West Fork. In the future, this may provide a good environment for on-foot exercise when visiting the region.[2]

There are also many nice short running loops in parks throughout the Dallas area, but they do not fit our formula.

* * * *

Dallas is a fascinating city to visit. Despite its apparent focus on automobiles, shops, business, and anything BIG, there are some very attractive aspects of life. First, the people are exceedingly friendly (until they get behind the wheel, that is). Second, there is a serious core of locals that really care about things like on-foot exercise. Third, there are two on-foot exercise routes, handy to downtown, that satisfy all of our criteria very well.

If you ever get the opportunity to spend a few days here in the heart of Texas, I have no doubt you'll enjoy some quality time out on-foot!

---

2       We learnt about the Campion Trails from Mike MacAllister's article at: http://www.dallasnews.com/sharedcontent/dallas/trails/campion.html

# 11

# Mile High City

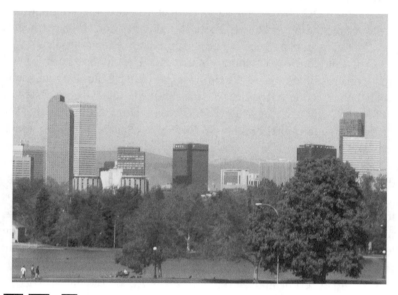

W here the Rockies meet the High Plains is where you find Denver, Colorado. Denver is a very outdoors-oriented city, due to at least three factors. First, there is the close proximity of the Rocky Mountains, which naturally engenders participation in such activities as hiking, skiing, mountaineering, and mountain biking. Second, there is an ideal climate for outdoors activities, with dry air, and nice temperatures most of the year. Third, there is a comparatively young population. Put these together and you get a relatively fit, outdoors-focused community, which is conscious about providing good on-foot exercise facilities in the city and throughout the region generally.

Denver's origins stem from the gold rush of the late 1850s. In 1858 William Green Russell discovered gold in what is now downtown Denver. More major discoveries in the front ranges quickly followed. The railroad arrived in 1870. In 1876, Colorado was admitted to the Union, with Denver its state capital. In the 1880s the focus shifted to the silver rush. In the Great Depression, Denver became Cow Town, thanks to its cattle feedlots that became the new way of fattening cattle. After World War II, the military and federal government moved in big time. Denver became the city with the most U.S. federal workers after Washington DC. More recently, Denver has become an important center of technology. This diversity of industries and skills permeates the city today, helping keep the population lively and youthful.

Denverites are serious sports enthusiasts. The city hosts teams in all major professional sports—the Broncos (NFL), the Colorado Avalanche (NHL), the Colorado Rockies (NL baseball), and the Nuggets (NBA).

Denver's moniker of Mile High City is literally accurate—the 13th step of the state capital building in Denver is exactly 5,280 feet above sea level.

As I noted earlier, Denver's weather is very good for outdoor exercise. The average maximum temperature is in our preferred 40-to-80 degrees range for nine months of the year, making it into the 80s in June, July, and August. There is precipitation on average 89 days per year—not a major concern. The air is generally very dry, meaning less sweating. Strenuous exercise is therefore more comfortable than in most cities.

The violent crime index is 6.2 (crimes per 1,000 residents in 2003)— close to the best for the cities we cover. (San Diego sneaks in better at 5.8, but compare these figures with Atlanta at 19.7.)

The Denver public transit system, operated by the Regional Transportation District (RTD), is a mixed bag for a visitor. There are two light rail lines that are immaculately clean and on time. Beyond that, one needs to depend on buses. There are many bus routes, but little system or organization—at least, that is how it seems to a visitor. For example, there are several express buses that generally only operate in limited hours, but the hours vary dramatically route-to-route. There is a paper system map, but the only places to get a copy seemed to be the Civic Center and Market Street bus stations. We found the RTD website a little difficult to use, but it does offer Colorado residents the opportunity to receive a free system map by mail.[1]

A major upgrade of the southeastern transportation corridor, called T-REX, is currently in development. We look forward to substantial improvements in the light rail services in that direction, scheduled for completion in 2006.[2]

\* \* \* \*

We had no difficulty finding on-foot routes in Denver, which is located on the confluence of the South Platte River and Cherry Creek. We successfully put together three excellent routes, which satisfy all of our criteria. It so happens that all of them start downtown and head off to other interesting points in greater Denver. (You could equally well do any of them in reverse; we shall discuss that alternative at the end.)

To keep life simple, we picked one nominal downtown start point for all routes—Colfax Avenue at Speer Boulevard, by the Colorado Convention Center. Colfax, which lays claim to being the longest continuous street in the United States, is as easy to find as Speer, which tracks Cherry Creek. This point is convenient to light rail lines, buses, and major downtown hotels.

| Route | Distance |
|---|---|
| 1. Inner Parks Loop | 7.3-to-9.5 miles |
| 2. South Platte River to Englewood | 9.6 miles |
| 3. Downtown to University of Denver | 5.2 miles |

---

1       See: http://www.rtd-denver.com/
2       See: http://www.trexproject.com/

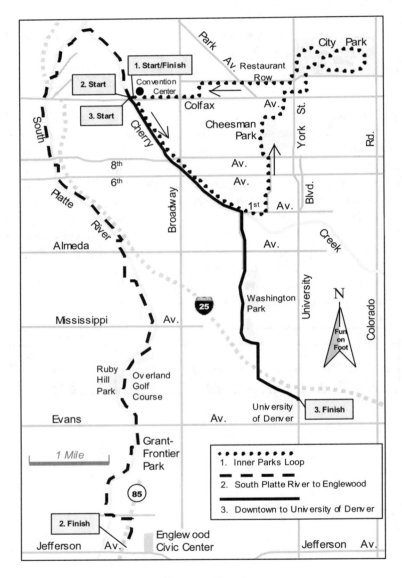

**Denver Routes**

# Inner Parks Loop

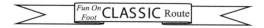

| Distance | 7.3-to-9.5 miles |
|---|---|
| Comfort | A mix of pedestrian/cyclist trails, pedestrian trails, and quality suburban streets. There are a few busy roads to cross at pedestrian lights, and the last 2.2-mile stretch back to downtown uses ordinary city sidewalks. The entire route is flat. Expect other pedestrian traffic around, even on quiet weekdays. |
| Attractions | A route with considerable variety, linking together: the Cherry Creek Greenway; a classy and attractive residential area; Cheesman Park; and Denver's largest urban park, City Park. There is bird life and some very attractive scenery in the parks. |
| Convenience | Start downtown near RTD light rail lines, the Civic Center Bus Station, the Convention Center, and downtown hotels. End either back downtown or at Restaurant Row (7.3 miles), where you can either walk or take a local bus back downtown. Total loop distance from/to the Convention Center is 9.5 miles. |
| Destination | Restaurant Row is one of Denver's most popular eating, drinking, and entertainment areas, with many choices for a wind-down spot; perfect for a post-run weekend brunch. Alternatively, complete the loop back to the start. |

This is one of the most interesting routes you will find anywhere. We have linked together three top-notch green spaces, all quite close to downtown. We have included a few blocks through a particularly attractive residential area, and made the end destination Denver's Restaurant Row where you have an enormous number of choices of eating and drinking places for a wind-down.

Start at our nominal downtown start point—Colfax Avenue at Speer Boulevard. A major advantage of this start point is that it is right on the Cherry Creek Greenway. The Greenway has a combined pedestrian

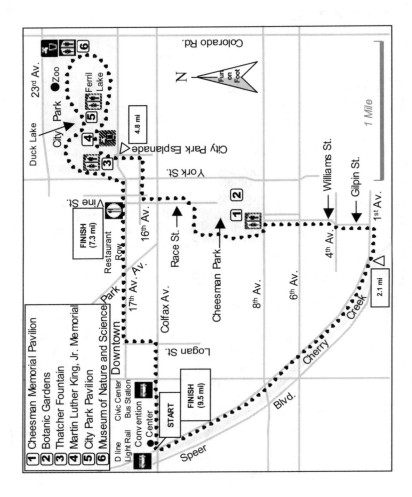

and bicycle trail, which follows the edge of Cherry Creek. It is sunken below street level, with no streets to cross—all the traffic passes above you.

From the Colfax-Speer intersection, take the steps down to the Greenway and then head south. There is a paved bike path with an unpaved foot trail adjacent for most of the way. Enjoy this trail, devoid of all automobile intrusions, for 2.1 miles. At that point the sunken trail ends and you should take the very last ramp up to street level—this brings you out on the south side of 1st Avenue.

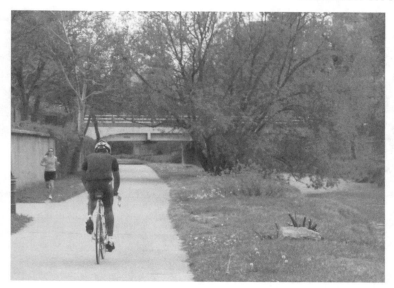

## Cherry Creek Greenway—Runners, Cyclists, and Instant Urban Escape

Proceed eastward on 1st Avenue, past the Colorado Country Club, to the traffic light at Gilpin Street. Cross 1st Avenue here and head northward up Gilpin Street. You find yourself in a very attractive residential neighborhood. There are wide, tree-lined streets, lovely homes, and little traffic. At 4th Avenue follow the dogleg into Williams Street, another quiet tree-lined street with more impressive homes. This leads you to Cheesman Park.

Cheesman Park, dedicated to the 19th century Denver businessman Walter Scott Cheesman, is a popular local green space frequented by many on-foot exercisers as well as picnickers, sunbathers, and others. Its centerpiece is the Grecian-style Cheesman Memorial Pavilion, built in 1910. The moderately trafficked roads through the park are not pedestrian-friendly. There is, however, a pedestrian path that roughly follows the park perimeter.

From Williams Street, you enter the park at its southern end. You need to get to its northeastern corner, so you can take your pick of the perimeter trail to the western side or the eastern side.

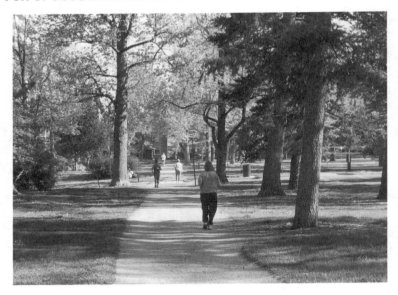

## Cheesman Park Perimeter Trail

At the northeast corner of the park, there is a laneway that takes you to 13th Avenue, near its intersection with Race Street. Head north on Race Street, a shady pleasant street, cross Colfax Avenue, and continue to 16th Avenue. There is some traffic here, but it is a relatively pedestrian-friendly area. At 16th Avenue turn right, heading eastwards. Cross busy York and Josephine Streets and proceed to the City Park Esplanade, where space, peace, and pleasantness start to unfold. The Esplanade is wide with grassy strips and little traffic. Turn left on the Esplanade, near the stately Denver East High School. After crossing 17th Avenue, you enter City Park, Denver's largest urban park with an area of 314 acres.

You soon come to the very impressive bronze and granite Thatcher Fountain, circa 1917. At this point, turn right on the pedestrian trail. Expect to find many other runners, walkers, mothers with babies, or people exercising dogs. Continue past the Martin Luther King, Jr. memorial, then the Pavilion. From this point, follow the shore of Ferril Lake, named after Thomas Hornsby Ferril, the 1979-1996 Poet Laureate of Colorado who wrote the poem *This Lake is Mine*, recalling the many times he walked his dog around this lake.

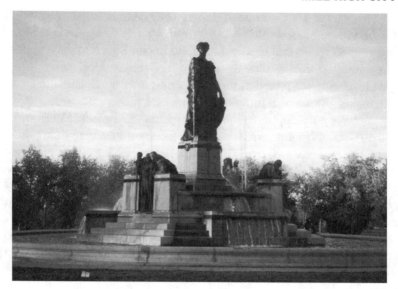

### Thatcher Fountain[3]

There is a collection of large buildings towards the northeast. These buildings comprise the Denver Museum of Nature and Science and the Gates Planetarium. There are various trails here. We suggest you proceed right up to the museum's back entrance to see the view, which combines the park's own beauty, the city skyline behind that, and the Rockies behind that. You might also wish to take advantage of the museum's restrooms, which are much more pleasant than the portable restrooms encountered elsewhere in Denver's parks. You can also get drinks and snacks. To get to these facilities, work your way around to the museum's north entrance (there is no charge to use these facilities).

After leaving the museum, continue around Ferril Lake, passing the Denver Zoo on your right. You come to Duck Lake on your right. (No prizes for guessing why it's called that.) On your left, if you are a fan of Robert Burns, Scotland's most famous poet, you will find a statue of him in a nice garden setting. Continue    following the trail westward, then towards the south without exiting the park. Go towards the southwest corner of the park where you'll find a park exit and a pedestrian crossing across busy York Street at 18th Avenue. After crossing, go one block south and turn right into 17th Avenue westbound.

---

3       Photo courtesy Western History Department, Denver Public Library

This part of 17th Avenue is known as Restaurant Row. You'll find the first restaurants starting a block from City Park at Gaylord Street and continuing several blocks through to Logan Street. A wide variety of cuisines is offered, plus there are a few conventional pubs. Most establishments are priced at the low to moderate level, and almost all will make customers in rumpled running gear feel comfortable.

We have put an optional route termination (7.3 miles) at Vine Street and 17th, for those readers who want a food and beverage destination. Here you find one of the best, all-round, eating and drinking places in the area, Rhino. Rhino has a creative menu for lunch and dinner daily, the food is very good, and the service is friendly. Saturday and Sunday brunch are also served. Despite several tries, I never received a good answer as to the source of the restaurant's name.

Restaurant Row continues several blocks to Logan Street. To continue on-foot to downtown, follow 17th Street to Logan, turn left into Logan, turn right into Colfax Avenue, and proceed past the State Capitol and Civic Center to the Convention Center. Alternatively, if you have had enough on-foot activity when you reach Restaurant Row, go a block north at any point to 18th Street, and catch the local bus downtown.

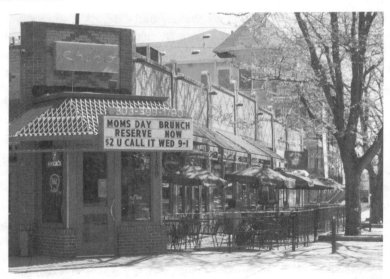

**Restaurant Row, Rhino Restaurant in Foreground**

# South Platte River to Englewood

| Distance | 9.6 miles |
|---|---|
| Comfort | A flat pedestrian/cyclist trail all the way. There is some other pedestrian or cyclist traffic around, even on quiet weekdays, but people may be sparse in a few parts. Crowds are unlikely. |
| Attractions | A range of different parkland environments, including the urban parks near downtown, the scenic confluence of the river with Cherry Creek, and various other parks and wildlife habitats distributed the length of the greenway. There are few automobile traffic encounters. |
| Convenience | Start downtown near RTD light rail lines, the Civic Center Bus Station, the Convention Center, and downtown hotels. End where you can catch a light rail service direct back to downtown. |
| Destination | Englewood City Center, a well-planned regional center with shops, entertainment, and at least one excellent eating and drinking establishment. |

The South Platte River is what originally attracted people to settle Denver—specifically, the small quantities of gold found there. (The gold veins in the nearby mountains soon proved a much more lucrative mining endeavor.) While the river was a neglected, polluted embarrassment for most of the city's life, for the past four decades a great deal of effort has been applied to cleaning it up and developing the South Platte River Greenway—a recreational and nature preserve. Today the river trail constitutes a well-formed and interesting on-foot exercise route.

Start at our usual downtown point, Colfax at Speer. Go down the steps to the Cherry Creek Greenway, but this time turn right heading downstream or northward. The path splits after Stout Street, with a pedestrian path on the east side of the creek and a bicycle path on the west side. Go roughly a mile to the confluence with the South Platte River. Here you find Confluence Park and Centennial Gardens, complete with year-round restrooms and water fountain. (The other restrooms marked on the map are seasonal.) Kayaking is popular around the confluence.

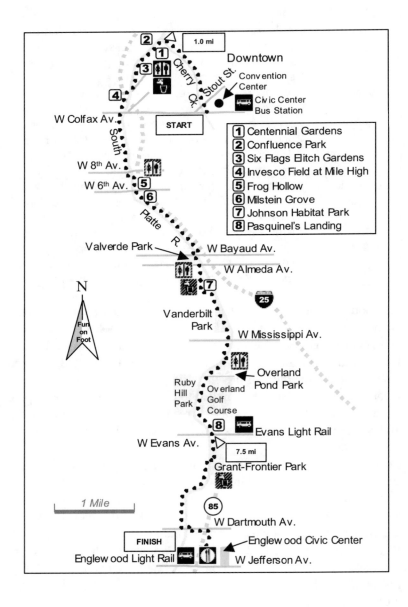

Downtown

Convention Center

Civic Center
Bus Station

W Colfax Av.

START

**1** Centennial Gardens
**2** Confluence Park
**3** Six Flags Elitch Gardens
**4** Invesco Field at Mile High
**5** Frog Hollow
**6** Milstein Grove
**7** Johnson Habitat Park
**8** Pasquinel's Landing

W 8th Av.

W 6th Av.

Valverde Park

W Bayaud Av.

W Almeda Av.

N

Fun on Foot

Vanderbilt Park

W Mississippi Av.

Overland Pond Park

Ruby Hill Park

Overland Golf Course

Evans Light Rail

W Evans Av.

7.5 mi

Grant-Frontier Park

1 Mile

85

W Dartmouth Av.

FINISH

Englewood Civic Center

Englewood Light Rail

W Jefferson Av.

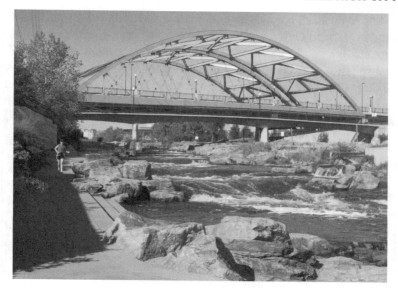

### The Confluence

From the confluence, follow the river upstream, which is southward. You can use either side of the river initially. Pass by the Six Flags Elitch Gardens amusement park. Then, if you are on the east bank of the river, you should cross to the west bank—near Invesco Field at Mile High, home of the Broncos.

Continue up the river. After crossing 8th Avenue, you come to a footbridge. Take that footbridge to the east bank. You now enter Frog Hollow Park, a recognized site of prehistoric civilization. Then pass through the park called Milstein Grove. Continue to the next footbridge, just north of Bayaud Avenue, and cross back to the west bank. The reserve here is called Valverde Park, not the prettiest of parks but the scenery improves as you move further south.

Pass through Johnson Habitat Park and Vanderbilt Park. These areas are under ongoing restoration so will undoubtedly become more pleasant in the future. Cross Mississippi Avenue. A little further on you come to another footbridge. Cross it back to the east bank. From this point on, you find a dramatic improvement in the scenic beauty of your surroundings.

You come to Overland Pond. This is a combined nature education area, picnic area, and fishing lake. It is very pleasant and you can expect to find many local families here. After that, the trail tracks the boundary of the Overland Golf Course, with very green, shady, and pleasant on-foot conditions. You come to the point called Pasquinel's Landing—you might be surprised to learn that this place does not celebrate the landing of a real person; rather it recognizes the colorful character Jacques Pasquinel in James Michener's epic novel, *Centennial*, that was set in Colorado. You then reach Evans Avenue.

---

**VARIATION**

Having gone 7.5 miles, you may have had enough on-foot exercise by now. If so, you can terminate the outing here. Take Evans Avenue eastward 0.3 mile to the Evans Station, where you can catch the Light Rail back downtown. There are some fast food outlets further along Evans, but not much else. Therefore, we encourage you to stay the course for another two miles to get to a more interesting and enjoyable destination.

---

A little south of Evans, you come to Grant-Frontier Park, the site of the first settlement in Denver, Montana City. It was established by miners in 1857. Cross the river at the footbridge.

Proceed along the river trail to Dartmouth Avenue, where we suggest you leave the river and head eastward. Cross to the south side of Dartmouth at the first pedestrian crossing. Then take the pedestrian/bicycle path towards the underpass under the rail tracks and Route 85. On exiting that underpass, turn right onto Inca street.

You are soon in the midst of total civilization, Englewood City Center. There are many shops (from Walmart down to tiny shops), fast foods, cinemas, and everything else you would expect to find in such a center. The one thing that took us a while to find was a good all-round eating and drinking establishment, in particular, one where we could feel comfortable in running gear. Eventually, after polling the locals, we found the answer—the Patriot and Loyalist Pub, on Inca Street close to Jefferson Avenue (Route 285). This place, a quite authentic British pub, was a real winner. The menu offered a choice of British pub food and American dishes. The food was excellent and the beer was cold.

The other good thing about the Patriot and Loyalist is that, when you leave it, you are just a few yards from the entrance to Englewood station. The Light Rail whisks you comfortably back to downtown.

---

# Downtown to University of Denver

| Distance | 5.2 miles |
|---|---|
| Comfort | Flat pedestrian/cyclist trails most of the way, with some short stretches on street sidewalks. Expect other pedestrian or cyclist traffic around, even on quiet weekdays. Crowds are unlikely. |
| Attractions | The Cherry Creek Greenway and Washington Park, one of Denver's most pleasant parks for on-foot exercisers. End at the University of Denver Campus. There are few automobile encounters. |
| Convenience | Start downtown near RTD light rail lines, the Civic Center Bus Station, the Convention Center, and downtown hotels. End where you can catch a bus back to downtown or walk 1.9 miles to a light rail station. (Light rail service directly from here is planned for December 2006.) |
| Destination | University of Denver campus, with a choice of campus-grade restaurants and pubs as wind-down spots. |

While this is a very pleasant route, it ranks a clear third in our selections. If you want to see the university campus, it will work great for you. Otherwise, you might find it a little lacking in terms of destination and the convenience of transport back downtown.

However, when Denver's T-REX transport expansion project is completed (targeted for December 2006), there will be a new University Boulevard light rail station right at the end of our route. At that point we expect this will become a winner route. Let us proceed with that expectation in mind…

Start at our usual downtown terminus, Colfax at Speer. Follow the Cherry Creek Greenway upstream as in our first route. However, this time, take the exit ramp to Downing Street. This ramp loops back onto Speer westbound. Turn immediately left into Downing Street and cross the creek via the bridge sidewalk. Then cross the Speer eastbound lanes at the light. You have now escaped the traffic!

Take the first left onto S Marion Parkway. Conditions for pedestrians become excellent now, with a wide tree-lined street, dedicated pedestrian path, and few vehicles. This street leads you to the northern entrance to Washington Park.

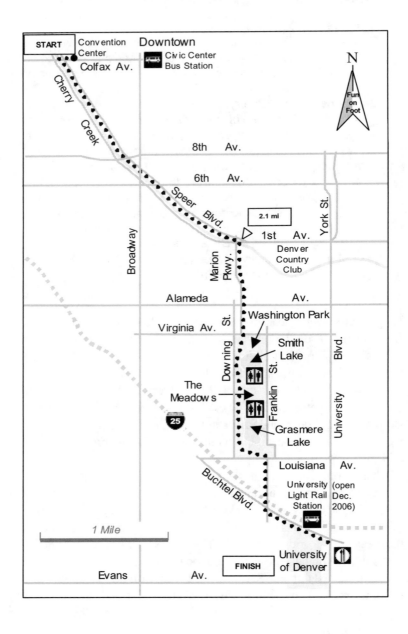

START

Convention Center

Colfax Av.

Downtown

Civic Center Bus Station

N

Fun on Foot

Cherry Creek

8th Av.

6th Av.

Speer Blvd.

Broadway

2.1 mi

1st Av.

York St.

Marion Pkwy.

Denver Country Club

Alameda Av.

Virginia Av.

Downing St.

Washington Park

Smith Lake

The Meadows

Franklin St.

Blvd.

University

25

Grasmere Lake

Louisiana Av.

Buchtel Blvd.

University Light Rail Station

(open Dec. 2006)

1 Mile

University of Denver

FINISH

Evans Av.

Enter the park and follow the road to the right. A major quality you will note is the absence of automobile through-traffic. Pass Smith Lake on your left and continue to a parking area. Then, in the right season, you pass an impressive set of flower gardens on your right. Cross one of the few remaining pieces of Smith's Ditch, Denver's first major irrigation channel whose construction started in 1860.

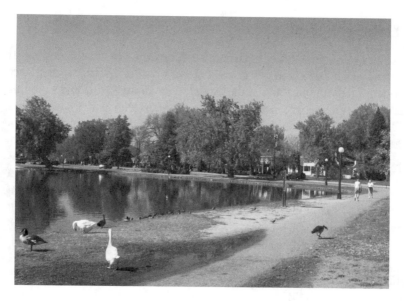

**Washington Park and its Plentiful Bird Life**

Pass the Meadow, a set of sporting fields, on your left. Then you come to Grasmere Lake, a popular fishing spot. You can go either way around Grasmere Lake. Whichever you choose, make your way to the southeastern corner of the park, and exit onto Louisiana Avenue. Find Franklin Street heading southbound.

Follow the sidewalk of Franklin Street across Interstate 25 then turn left on Buchtel Boulevard. Continue to University Boulevard, or peel off southward if you have particular campus destinations in mind.

The intersection of Buchtel and University is a good reference point for terminating our route. If you want to see the campus, it is directly south from here. If you want a meal or drink, there are one or two acceptable places nearby on University Boulevard, or other places on Evans Avenue (go two blocks south, then head westward on Evans).

When the T-REX project is complete, you will find a light rail station here on Buchtel, west of University).

Prior to completion of T-REX, the simplest way to get back downtown is to take a local bus north on University Boulevard. Alternatively, walk 1.9 miles; first south to Evans Avenue then west along Evans to the Evans light rail station. Admittedly, neither option is ideal.

# Other Ideas

Any of our above three routes can be done in the reverse direction. If that works for you, you will be treated to a selection of interesting places to wind-down your route in the downtown vicinity. Nola and I did this a couple of times and became attached to Pints Pub at 13th Avenue and Cherokee Street. It is about a quarter-mile from our nominal downtown termination point of Colfax and Speer, two blocks south and four blocks east. It is handy to the Civic Center.

Pints Pub is a traditional British brewpub—as traditional as you could ever expect to find in the United States. It boasts two special features. First, it is the purveyor of the largest selection of single-malt whiskies outside of Edinburgh, Scotland. Second, it brews traditional British handcrafted "cask-conditioned" or "live" ales served via hand-pump—something very rare in the United States. Regardless of whether these features turn you on, if you are at all partial to the British pub concept, you should enjoy the food and excellent company here.

There are also many eating, drinking, and entertainment spots in the lower downtown (LoDo) area and around Coors Field, northwest of central downtown. Or you may just find your favorite place elsewhere…

One impressive route that we have not filled out is the continuation of the **Cherry Creek Greenway** south of 1st Avenue. Despite the need to divert to the streets around the Denver Country Club (thumbs down to the DCC for this unreasonableness!), the continuation of the route from the Cherry Creek Shopping Center onwards is a popular on-foot exercise route with locals. We omitted this route because we just could not find a suitably compelling destination point and convenient public transit back downtown. However, should you be living in, staying in, or heading to somewhere handy to the Cherry Creek corridor as far south as the Cherry Creek Reservoir (Cherry Creek Dam Road), consider using the Greenway.

The **Denver Technology Center** is about two miles southwest of Cherry Creek Reservoir, roughly ten miles south of downtown Denver. Undoubtedly, many visitors to town will end up staying near there. It offers its own pleasant on-foot environment, with interlinking paths, many with colorful flowerbeds and trees, built into the landscape design of the entire development. Furthermore, the T-REX project plans to service that area with light rail transit. When that is complete, it will open up a very attractive on-foot route between downtown Denver and the Technology Center, via the Cherry Creek Greenway. We look forward to this option coming available.

While we have specifically targeted Denver because of its status as a major U.S. city, we feel we should also draw attention to some other nearby Colorado cities. In particular, both Colorado Springs and Boulder were named in *Runner's World's* 2002 "10 Best Running Cities."[4] If you find yourself staying in either of those places, be sure to take the opportunity to explore and exercise on-foot.

On that note, we shall finish up our coverage of Denver and the mountain states. Enjoy the Rockies and what is nearby! Next we head to the final western frontier—the Pacific coast and its character-filled major cities: Seattle, San Francisco, Los Angeles, and San Diego…

---

4       See: http://www.runnersworld.com/article/0,5033,s6-188-0-0-1199-1-4X7-3,00.html

# 12

# The Emerald City

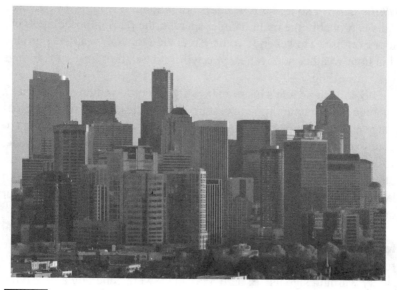

T he history of Western civilization in the Seattle region began in 1792 when Captain Vancouver explored and named Puget Sound. Western settlement started in 1851 with the arrival of a party led by David Denny. They met Native American leader Chief Seattle, the man to be honored later in the naming of this city. Treaties were subsequently signed with most local Native American tribal leaders and, despite some early hiccups, a comparatively stable settlement was well on the way by the 1860's.

Seattle today—home to Boeing, Microsoft, Starbucks, and Amazon. com—is a major center of modern U.S. industry. Seattle also has a character and style that is easy to embrace. To us Canadians, Seattle has a Canadian feel about it. It has mountains and skiing nearby. It is laid back, comparatively young, and very outdoors oriented. It has loads of salmon, crabs, and other seafood. And—you will quickly notice—strangers greet each other in the street.

Seattle is also the proud winner of the 2005 Fittest City award from *Men's Fitness* magazine. According to the magazine's research, 85% of Seattle residents claim to get at least *some* exercise every month, and the city has better-than-average air quality, tons of gyms and sporting goods stores, and great access to outdoor recreation.[1]

There is only one significant negative factor about Seattle: *it rains all the time* (or so it seems). If it is not raining, it is foggy or overcast. This is probably the main damper (pardon the pun) imposed upon on-foot exercise. However, if you are prepared to work your way around this little weather annoyance, you will find Seattle's on-foot offerings very rewarding.

Looking at Seattle's historical weather record, we find that the city's average daily maximum temperature is in our desired 40-to-80 degrees range all year round. So temperature is unlikely to be an impediment to your exercising outdoors at any time. However, there are, on average, 150 rainy days per year—41% of all days. Also, compared with most other U.S. cities, Seattle's high latitude causes it to get dark early from late fall through to early spring. Take this fact into account in your outdoor exercise scheduling.

As to safety, Seattle's violent crime index is 6.8 (crimes per 1,000 residents in 2003), among the best figures for cities we visited. On the routes we cover, and other routes we investigated, we saw no major safety warning signals. In particular, there were generally ample other pedestrians or cyclists around. However, always use appropriate common-sense precautions.

Seattle residents are largely dependent on the automobile for many aspects of life, in particular for commuting between downtown and such centers as Bellevue, Redmond, and points south. In fact, it is very compelling to have a car just to get to and from the Seattle-Tacoma Airport. The freeway system around Seattle is very heavily loaded. The good news, though, is that the traffic does not encroach very seriously into the downtown streets or the areas that are most attractive for on-foot exercise.

---

1        Jeff Lucia, "7th Annual Report: America's Fittest & Fattest Cities 2005," *Men's Fitness*, February 2005.

If you are staying in or near downtown, you can get to and from all routes we suggest either on-foot or via the bus system (the King County Metro). However, unless you are already familiar with that bus system, be prepared for a few inherent hazards in it.

The bus network has excellent coverage, and is generally clean and tidy. Beyond those laudable points, after first using the system I became convinced that its designers were going out of their way to outdo the New York Subway folk on the degree of confusion and chaos imposed on visitors to town.

Here are a few examples of problems:

- There are hundreds of routes, and service frequencies vary anywhere from 15 minutes to an hour, even on weekdays. Saturday and Sunday coverage varies anywhere from none to same-as-weekdays.
- Guidance is scarce. While bus stops have a route number posted, there are no further clues as to route geography, frequency, or schedule. The only way to know when a bus is scheduled is to have a paper timetable, obtained either on the bus (not much use for a first-time user) or at the King Street or Westlake Customer Service Office (if you can find one of them). We suggest you print timetables in advance from the Metro website.
- There is a paper *Transit Map & Rider's Guide*, but the only places to obtain one seem to be the two Customer Service Offices. Unfortunately, this guide fails to answer most questions as to the best route to take from *A* to *B*. You need the route maps in the timetables too.
- The folk who wrote the *Transit Map & Rider's Guide* have curious communication skills. For example, it brightly informs cyclists that, "All Metro buses are equipped with bicycle racks." Sounds great! It then qualifies that nice message, with, "Bicycles may be loaded or unloaded at any bus stop at any time, except in the Ride Free Area between 6 a.m. and 7 p.m. During these hours, loading/unloading bikes is restricted to a route's first and last ride free stop and the tunnel stops at Convention Place and the International District." I felt real good that I was not a cyclist!
- The fare system is even more confusing. In particular, you sometimes pay when you get on the bus and sometimes when you

get off. It does not take a brilliant intellect to realize that expecting people to pay when they get off a bus is not a very good idea. When we took a bus to the university, absolutely every student, when disembarking, looked surprised and told the driver, "Sorry, I don't have any money." There's not much the poor driver can do at this point except scowl and say, "Get off!"

- Fares and ticket requirements vary according to zone and time of day. If you are sporadic in your use of the system I recommend carrying around a stock of quarters and singles to pay fares.

- Finally, note one surprising positive feature of the system. When you get on (or maybe off) a bus the driver might offer you a little slip of paper. Don't underestimate its value. It is a lottery ticket that you should present to every other bus driver all day, and will entitle you to free travel anywhere in the system for a mystery period from two to eight hours.

\* \* \* \*

What makes Seattle a number one location for interesting and attractive on-foot exercise routes is the region's fascinating geography, with far more than its fair share of water features including ocean inlets, rivers, and lakes.

We tried several routes in and around the urban area and finally settled on four routes, all of which satisfy our criteria. There are also opportunities to link and mix these routes. We hope you enjoy these routes like we did!

| Route | Distance |
|-------|----------|
| 1.  Discovery Park to Downtown | 8.9 miles |
| 2.  Green Lake and Fremont | 4.4 miles |
| 3.  The Arboretum and Lake Washington | 4.0-to-6.0 miles |
| 4.  Burke-Gilman Trail to Ballard | 7.1 miles |

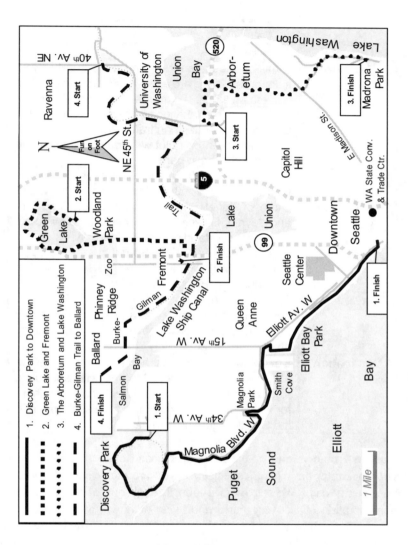

**Seattle Routes**

# Discovery Park to Downtown

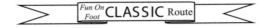

| | |
|---|---|
| **Distance** | 8.9 miles |
| **Comfort** | A mix of pedestrian trails and good quality street sidewalks. There are a few busy roads to cross at pedestrian lights. There are some grades to deal with, so it might take longer than you would think. Expect other pedestrian traffic around on most of the route, even on quiet weekdays. Not suitable for inline skating in parts. |
| **Attractions** | Do a loop through Seattle's Discovery Park, with its varied-terrain nature trails. Then follow the shore of Puget Sound, through Elliott Bay Park and Myrtle Edwards Park back to downtown. There are outstanding views of the city, its docks, its surrounds, and Puget Sound, on the way. On arriving downtown, follow the waterfront to the Aquarium and Pike Place Market. |
| **Convenience** | To start, take a number 19, 24, or 33 Metro bus from 4th Avenue downtown to Discovery Park. End downtown convenient to restaurants, entertainment, and hotels. |
| **Destination** | Downtown Seattle. We nominally terminate the route at the Pike Place Market, with shopping, sightseeing, and some excellent restaurant/bars for winding down. Downtown hotels, shops, and the Seattle Aquarium are nearby. |

Our first route is one of the most scenic and enjoyable routes you will encounter anywhere, especially if you are lucky enough to do it on a sunny day. We start with a loop through one of Seattle's most popular parks, Discovery Park, northwest of downtown. This 534-acre wilderness park has terrain that varies from old growth forests to open bluff-top paths with spectacular views. We then tack on a glorious scenic route along Puget Sound, terminating in downtown Seattle.

We nominally start at the Discovery Park visitor center, just inside the West Government Way entrance to the park. To get there from downtown by public transit, catch a Metro bus in 4th Avenue,

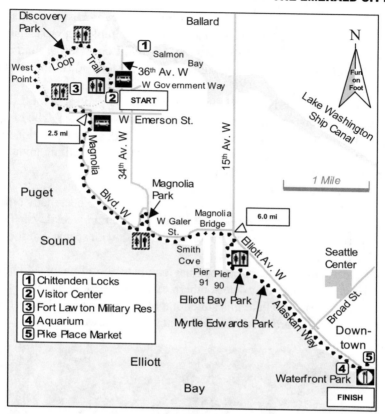

with destination Discovery Park. When we last did this, there were three such bus routes—numbers 19, 24, and 33—and each one was sufficiently infrequent that you have to be prepared to accept any one of them. This reduces your maximum wait time to 20 minutes. King County Metro always likes creating little challenges for its riders, and the one here is that the different bus routes go to different places. The number 19 and 24 buses terminate at the park's southern gate. Enter the park and head northeast following the signs to the Loop Trail. It is 0.3 mile to the visitor center. If, however, you scored the number 33 bus, get off at the 36th Avenue stop (on W Government Way), enter the park there, and then follow the signs to the visitor center. A good reason to go to the visitor center is to pick up a map, and there are also restrooms. However, note that the visitor center is closed on Mondays and any day remotely resembling a holiday.

There are many paths and various things to see in Discovery Park, so choose any route that takes your fancy. The simplest approach, and a very rewarding one, is to follow the 2.8-mile Loop Trail around the park. The Loop Trail can be picked up on the western side of the visitor center.

Discovery Park is well signposted, so it is easy to track the Loop Trail and understand the optional attractions on its offshoots. The Loop Trail is soft underfoot and bicycles are prohibited, so this is a runners' and walkers' paradise. It traverses beautiful forest terrain initially, opening out into grassy fields later.

There are some modest grades, but nothing particularly steep. We were there in late fall and the colors were stunning. Expect many other on-foot folk there, both runners and walkers, even on weekdays. The southernmost part of the trail traverses cliff-tops, with scenic overlooks of Puget Sound.

Proceed around the trail, circumnavigating the Fort Lawton Military Reservation. Continue to the southern exit of the park, which leads to W Emerson Street. Take this street one block eastward to the start of Magnolia Boulevard W. This heads you towards downtown.

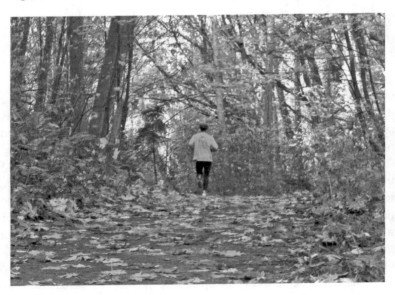

**Discovery Park's Loop Trail**

Magnolia Boulevard W is a lightly trafficked road with a good sidewalk and its fair share of on-foot exercisers. The first few blocks are residential suburbia. However, after a while the road joins up with the cliff-top, with views of Puget Sound and magnificent homes above and below.

---

**VARIATION**

As an alternative to the first part of Magnolia Boulevard W, if you feel a little adventurous and would like to follow a secluded traffic-free road through attractive waterfront homes, head westward two blocks on W Emerson Street and turn left into Perkins Lane West. This winding narrow street takes you down and along a level roughly halfway up the cliffs. Follow it to its end, where there are steps up to Magnolia Boulevard West. Be warned that the steps are many and steep.

---

Follow Magnolia Boulevard W until it takes a hard turn left. Continue following it to its subsequent bend to the right and across a bridge over a ravine. The road then bends back to the right and you come to Magnolia Park—a nice rest spot for a break, should you need one, with restrooms (open in summer only).

Keep following the road above the cliffs. It changes name to W Galer Street and then leads you to the Magnolia Bridge. This bridge provides an exhilarating downhill run or jog, with world-winning views of busy Piers 88 through 91 and a Seattle skyline backdrop.

The bridge brings you to Elliott Avenue W. Keep following the pedestrian sidewalk hard to the right, one short block to a cyclist/pedestrian ramp. This ramp takes you up to a path along a vehicle overpass over the rail tracks.

At this point you are eight miles from the route's start at the Discovery Park visitor center. If you are feeling tired, take heart, since the rest of the route is on flat, dedicated trails along the shore, generally away from automobile traffic. Furthermore, you can expect to be in the company of many Seattle locals out for their regular on-foot workout.

As you exit the overpass, continue bearing right on the pedestrian path. You come to a dedicated cyclist and pedestrian trail, with the sign "Pier 91 Bike Trail." Turn left onto the trail heading southward.

---

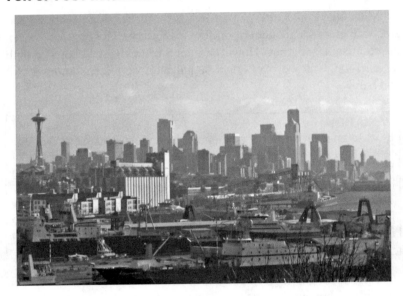

**The View from Magnolia Bridge**

After a short distance, the trail turns 90 degrees to the left and you enter Elliott Bay Park. The trail here splits into separate bicycle and pedestrian paths, and there are restrooms and water fountains.

After Elliott Bay Park ends, Myrtle Edwards Park starts. The pedestrian trail is outstanding in quality right through to Broad Street, at the Waterfront Streetcar's northern terminus.

---

**VARIATION**

At Broad Street, you have the opportunity to leave the waterfront and access the nearby Seattle Center or the north end of downtown. The Seattle Center, distinguished by the famous Space Needle, is the site of the 1962 *Century 21* World's Fair. We found a very good Irish Pub nearby—T.S. McHugh's in Mercer Street at 1st Avenue. It offered good food and ale, and is ideal for winding down from eight miles of exercise. Alternatively, you can ride the streetcar further downtown if that is your destination and you have had enough on-foot action by now.

---

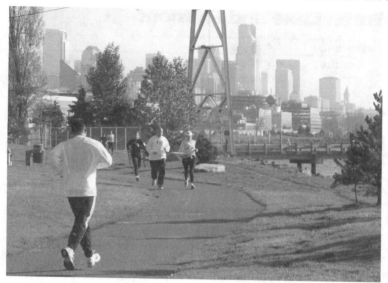

### Elliott Bay Park

To continue on-foot, keep on the waterfront-side sidewalk of Alaskan Way. You can expect substantial pedestrian traffic, with automobile traffic nearby, but at least there is no cross-traffic.

Our nominal end point is Pike Street, near the Seattle Aquarium. You can choose to see the Aquarium, or head inland, up the Pike Street Hillclimb. This takes you to the Pike Place Market, with its wide array of shopping options and some excellent nearby eating and drinking establishments. Pike Street Market was established in 1907.

If you are anything like Nola and me, you'll be more than ready for some food and a cold drink after finishing this exciting, but somewhat challenging, nine-mile route. We hunted out Kells Irish Restaurant and Pub in Post Alley, widely recognized as one of Seattle's best Irish establishments. We were not disappointed. It is a cozy place that serves an excellent lunch, including creative salads and traditional Irish favorite entrees. There are several other fine eating-places around here as well.

You have also ended at a place very convenient to the main downtown hotels, shops, and public transit.

# Green Lake and Fremont

| | |
|---|---|
| **Distance** | 4.4 miles |
| **Comfort** | A mix of pedestrian trails and good quality street sidewalks. There are a few roads to cross at pedestrian lights. The route is flat or downhill. There is other pedestrian traffic around on most of the route, even on quiet weekdays. Mostly OK for inline skating. |
| **Attractions** | Do a loop of attractive and popular Green Lake. Connect via Woodland Park and street sidewalks to Fremont, one of Seattle's most lively restaurant and tourist areas. |
| **Convenience** | To start, take a number 16 Metro bus from 3$^{rd}$ Avenue downtown (or 5$^{th}$ Avenue at the Seattle Center) to Woodlawn Avenue, near Green Lake. End at Fremont with convenient bus service back downtown from Fremont Avenue at N 34$^{th}$ Street. |
| **Destination** | Fremont, one of Seattle's most lively shop-browsing, restaurant, and entertainment areas. There are some excellent wind-down places here. You can catch a bus back downtown or, if you want to do another three-to-four miles on-foot, walk or run via the western edge of Lake Union. |

The 2.8-mile loop around Green Lake is Seattle's most popular on-foot trail, for runners, walkers, strollers, and dog-walkers alike. Our route includes that loop, and tacks on a short distance to Fremont, a great wind-down area. From Fremont you can get back downtown either by bus or on-foot.

Our suggested start point for this route is the intersection of Woodlawn Avenue N and Kirkwood Place N, the first Green Lake bus stop on the number 16 Metro bus route. This bus has a respectable 20-minute frequency. The number 26 bus also goes to the lake but it is less frequent.

Make your way northward to the lakeshore. Head counterclockwise around the lake trail. Expect to find many local runners, walkers, inline skaters, and cyclists on this trail. There is a wide paved path, with separate lanes for people on foot and people on wheels.

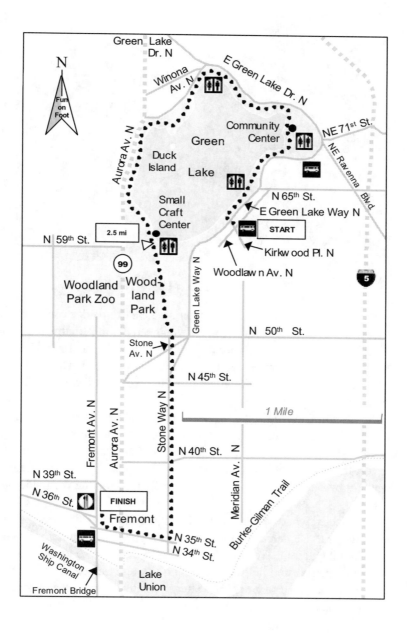

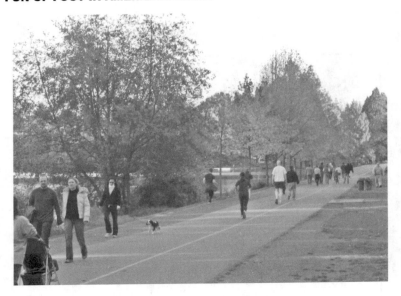

### The Popular Green Lake Trail

You come to the Community Center on the eastern edge of the lake. There are restrooms and water, should you need them. Continue north. At 0.8 mile from the Community Center you pass the Bath House Theater (there are no public facilities here). Then pass the Duck Island Game Reserve. At the southern end of the lake, pass the Small Craft Center and Aqua Theater.

At this point, we suggest you leave the lakeshore and head south into Woodland Park. There are various ways through this park. However, the ability to wander at will through the park is severely hampered by the fact that the noisy highway known variously as Aurora Avenue or Route 99 bisects it. It also is somewhat hilly towards the west side of the park.

We selected what we think is the easiest way through the park. After the Small Craft Center, cross the main road. There is an entrance drive into a parking area in Woodland Park. Follow this drive to the tennis courts and the sporting fields. There is no through-vehicle traffic here. Continue through the park to N 50th Street, passing through an enormous local sporting and recreation area.

Cross N 50th Street and find Stone Avenue N. Follow that street southward. Cross Green Lake Way. This brings you into a mainly residential area. The road is wide here, the sidewalks are good, and vehicle traffic is light. Around N 45th Street there are some eating and drinking places but we suggest continuing downhill a bit further. Keep on Stone Way N. Don't follow the road traffic where it diverts on Bridge Way towards the Aurora Avenue car-zoo.

Continue on Stone to N 35th Street. Turn right there and go a few short blocks, over a short rise, and emerge in civilization at Fremont Avenue in the middle of Fremont's pulsing heart. There are at least a dozen great restaurant/bars within a block of here, along with various trendy shops.

We liked Dad Watsons Restaurant and Brewery in Fremont Avenue at N 36th Street. They have a good variety of food, with a specialty in southern dishes. Drinks included the house's microbrews. There is also a quaint English Pub, the George and Dragon, a few blocks west on N 36th Street, with genuine English pub food.

You can take the number 26 or 28 bus from Fremont back downtown. Catch the bus on the west side of Fremont Avenue at N 34th Street.

---

**VARIATION**

If you feel like running or walking another three-to-four miles back to downtown, cross the Fremont Bridge and go south around the western edge of Lake Union. At the south end of the lake, continue to your desired destination via city streets. Alternatively, at the Fremont Bridge you intersect the Burke-Gilman trail, so you have an opportunity to link up with our fourth route.

---

# The Arboretum and Lake Washington

| | |
|---|---|
| **Distance** | 4.0-to-6.0 miles |
| **Comfort** | Mainly dedicated pedestrian trails plus some good quality street sidewalks. The route has some grades. There are minimal intrusions from automobile or bicycle traffic. There is other pedestrian traffic around on most of the route, even on quiet weekdays. Not suitable for inline skating. |
| **Attractions** | Follow the Arboretum Waterfront Trail through unique wetlands terrain, pass through the Washington Park Arboretum, and then connect with the shore of Lake Washington. |
| **Convenience** | To start, take any of several possible buses to the Montlake Freeway Station. (From downtown, a good choice is the number 43 Metro bus from Pike Street.) End on the Lake Washington Shore at a point with a bus service back downtown. |
| **Destination** | The Lake Washington Shore, very pleasant and with convenient public transit back downtown. Unfortunately there are no suitable eating-drinking wind-down places on the lakeshore. Rather, take the bus to a suitable wind-down establishment downtown or near the Seattle center. You can select your own actual termination point. We nominally terminate our 4.0-mile route at Madrona Park where there is a 15-minute bus service downtown. If you have the time and patience, extend the route another one or two miles to Leschi Park or Colman Park, where bus services run on more like a 30-minute schedule. |

This is an extremely attractive route. Start in the Montlake area at the southern end of the Montlake Bridge. By public transit, take any bus that stops at the Montlake Freeway Station. From downtown, the best service is the 15-minute number 43 bus caught in Pike Street. From the Montlake Freeway Station, follow the right-hand sidewalk of Montlake Boulevard E north towards the bridge. Before the bridge, take the narrow path and steps down to near the water level. Here you find the Lake Washington Ship Canal Waterside Trail. Follow it eastward,

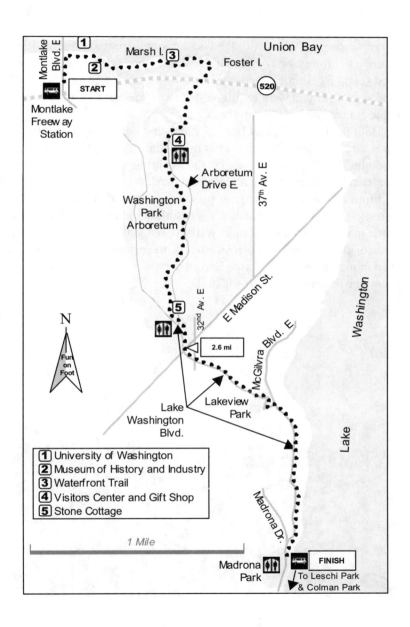

Union Bay

Montlake Blvd. E

Marsh I. ③

② Foster I.

START

520

Montlake Freeway Station

④

Arboretum Drive E.

37th Av. E

Washington Park Arboretum

N

Fun on Foot

⑤

32nd Av. E

E Madison St.

Washington

2.6 mi

McGilvra Blvd. E

Lake Washington Blvd.

Lakeview Park

Lake

① University of Washington
② Museum of History and Industry
③ Waterfront Trail
④ Visitors Center and Gift Shop
⑤ Stone Cottage

1 Mile

Madrona Dr.

Madrona Park

FINISH

To Leschi Park & Colman Park

passing the Husky Stadium across the canal, to just below the Museum of History and Industry (MOHAI), where the Arboretum Waterfront Trail starts.

Traversing the Waterfront Trail is a quite amazing experience. It is a nature trail through one of Seattle's few remaining wetland areas. It has been set up by Seattle's Department of Parks and Recreation as a self-guided tour. If you want to follow that tour, you can pick up a printed guide at nearby MOHAI for a nominal charge.

Both the bird and plant life are interesting here—especially if you are a city dweller. The construction of the trail is also interesting, involving a mix of floating walks, linking bridges, and soft paths over two islands—Marsh Island and Foster Island.

From the on-foot exerciser's perspective, you might want to walk in some parts, in deference to the possible damage you might cause to the trail or to yourself should you slip, but generally it is a flat, soft surface, ideal for the on-footer. Certainly, there are no cars, bicycles, or even inline skates around here. Expect to pass other on-foot exercisers, every one wearing an ear-to-ear smile.

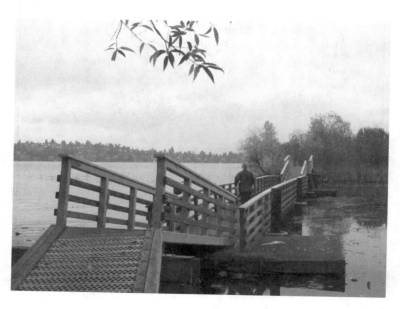

**The Arboretum Waterfront Trail**

Follow the waterfront trail to its end on Foster Island, and there pick up the Foster Point Trail heading inland to the Arboretum. It takes you under the Route 520 freeway via an underpass, and subsequently over a footbridge to the mainland, near the golf clubhouse. Continue a short distance to the entrance to the Arboretum and the sign heralding the Donald S. Graham Visitors Center. Pick up a free map here, and use the restroom if needed. We found the volunteer people here enormously helpful and friendly.

It is an excellent Arboretum—very attractive with widely varied plant life—and admission is free. It is very popular with on-foot exercisers, for good reason. There is a choice of north-to-south trails through the park, including two roads—Arboretum Drive E, which has few cars but some bicycles, and the busier Lake Washington Boulevard. We suggest following Arboretum Drive E and the various side trails near it—these side trails are generally more beautiful and cyclists are barred from them.

When we were in the Arboretum in the fall, the colors were outstanding. We are used to great fall colors in New England, but the display here was just as impressive, with an excellent variety of trees.

Pick your own trail southward to the Arboretum's south exit where Arboretum Drive E meets Lake Washington Boulevard. Pass the Stone Cottage. There is a restroom across the road here.

Exit the Arboretum and continue onwards to the Lake Washington shore via some beautiful residential areas.

Follow Lake Washington Boulevard east to Madison Street, cross that street, and continue straight ahead. At 32nd Avenue it becomes a bit confusing. Keep following the main road but, since there is no sidewalk for a short distance, take a pedestrian path to the left or an access road to the right, either of which eventually brings you back to Lake Washington Boulevard.

Continue on to Lakeview Park. There are some major downhill doglegs in the road here. Pedestrians can find shortcuts through the doglegs. After Lakeview Park, there are various routes to the lakeshore, down quite a substantial vertical drop. Pick whatever works for you.

Work your way down and continue south to Madrona Park, a pleasant park with restrooms, 4.0 miles from our start at the Montlake Freeway Station. We nominally terminate our route here because it is at the terminus of the number 2 bus route, which offers a frequent (15-

minute) service back downtown. If you are not in a hurry and want to do a couple more miles, read the variation below.

---

**VARIATION**

Continue further south along the Lake Washington shore. Go roughly one further mile to Leschi Park (there are restrooms here) and optionally another mile to Colman Park. From points between these two parks you can catch a number 27 bus back downtown, with a roughly 30-minute service. Alternatively, you can continue a further three miles to Seeward Park, and catch the number 34 bus.

---

There are no notable eating or drinking establishments on the lakeshore around here, but the number 2 bus can take you to many good places—either downtown or near the Seattle Center.

# Burke-Gilman Trail to Ballard

| | |
|---|---|
| **Distance** | 7.1 miles |
| **Comfort** | The Burke-Gilman Trail is a paved pedestrian/ cyclist trail, with soft pedestrian side-paths much of the way. We tack on 0.8 miles, via street sidewalks, to take you to the center of Ballard. The route is flat throughout, and there are no major traffic encounters. Expect other pedestrian traffic on the Burke-Gilman trail, even on quiet weekdays. Ballard streets have some quieter sections but there are usually other people around. Generally OK for inline skating. |
| **Attractions** | Enjoy a quality urban trail, traverse the University of Washington campus, follow the north shore of Lake Union and the Lake Washington Ship Canal, and see popular Gas Works Park. End in the historic and character-filled Ballard area. |
| **Convenience** | To start, take a number 74 Metro bus (roughly 30-minute service) from the Seattle Center to access the Burke-Gilman trail on the northeast side of the University District. There are also options to travel on-foot from downtown. End at Ballard, where you can catch the number 17 or 18 bus (each roughly a 30-minute service) back downtown. |
| **Destination** | Ballard, a Seattle precinct with a fishing, seafaring, and Scandinavian heritage. There are various restaurants, pubs, and interesting sights, including the Chittenden Locks and fish ladder, and the Nordic Heritage Museum. |

The Burke-Gilman Trail is an outstanding resource for outdoor exercisers in Seattle. It is a paved trail, extending over 14 miles from Kenmore, north of Seattle on the Lake Washington shore, to precincts close to the city. We decided to restrict our coverage to the city end of the trail, convenient to the urban transit network. The western end of the trail is near the interesting urban neighborhood of Ballard, which we made our nominal destination.

The Burke-Gilman trail is not the easiest place to get by public transit, but there is a reasonable bus service (roughly 30-minute, seven days a week) from the Seattle Center to the University District's

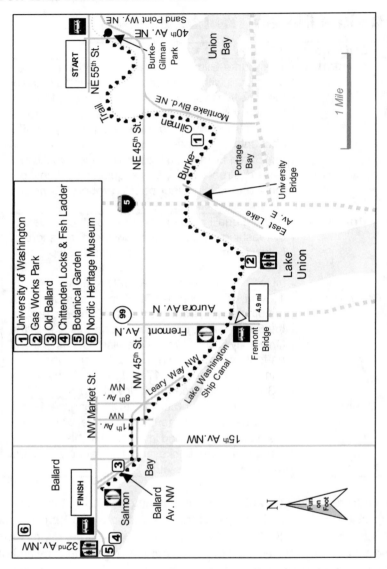

northeast corner. Catch the number 74 bus at its terminus at 1st Avenue N and Republican Street. Alight on NE 55th Street near 40th Avenue NE, and go south to pick up the trail. Follow the trail southwest. You get to experience some very pleasant parts of the trail, as it snakes through the University of Washington campus and its surrounds.

Where the trail goes under the University Bridge, you leave the university precinct and start to follow the northern edge of Lake Union and the Lake Washington Ship Canal. We found this trail very colorful in fall.

---

**VARIATION**

If you don't like buses and/or universities, you can start your route at the southern end of Lake Union. You can get there quickly on foot from downtown, via Westlake Avenue. Then follow the eastern edge of Lake Union (East Lake Avenue E and/or Fairview Avenue E) to the University Bridge, where you pick up the trail. Depending on just where you started downtown, this variation of the route is roughly the same distance as our nominal route. It is not enormously attractive, but does have some interesting sights, such as seaplane docks and Lake Union's on-water residences.

---

Follow the Burke-Gilman Trail to Gas Works Park. This is an attractive park, popular for family picnicking and activities such as kite flying. Continue along the trail to the Fremont Bridge.

---

**VARIATION**

If five miles is enough for you, you can exit the Burke-Gilman trail at the Fremont Bridge and enjoy the wind-down offerings of Fremont (as discussed in our second route). From Fremont, there is a frequent bus service downtown, or you can head there on-foot via the west shore of Lake Union.

---

We suggest you continue to the end of the Burke-Gilman Trail, and then on to Ballard, adding another 2.2 miles from Fremont.

Towards the end of the trail, the route becomes a little confusing. Keep following the pedestrian path near the rail tracks. The trail ends officially at 11th Avenue NW and NW 45th Street.

At this point, you need to make your way westward via local streets. The easiest approach is to take 11th Avenue north and turn left on NW Leary Way. Cross 15th Avenue NW, the busy street feeding the Ballard Bridge. At the next street—17th Avenue NW—Leary changes names to Leary Avenue NW. Turn left and go one block south to Ballard Avenue NW, the main street of what is known unofficially as *Old Ballard.*

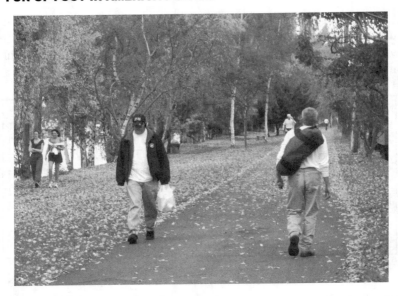

## The Burke-Gilman Trail by the Lake Washington Ship Canal

Old Ballard looks a bit run-down, but it has enormous character. It seems this part of Ballard was let slip downhill for several years, as the center of commerce drifted a couple of blocks north to NW Market Street. However, the tide has now started to turn and one can see signs of Old Ballard becoming a trendy area, with its own tourist appeal.

We nominally terminate our route in the heart of Ballard, where Ballard Avenue NW meets NW Market Street. Nola and I ate at down-home Hattie's Hat Restaurant in Ballard Avenue NW. We had a very enjoyable brunch there, and a good chat with some of the locals. However, be prepared for a slightly eccentric, rather than mainstream, culture around these parts.

Ballard's unique appeal stems from its early days as a fishing and seafaring town, and a center of Scandinavian immigration. Today, Scandinavian cultural traditions are still very evident, and Ballard is host to several Scandinavian festivals throughout the year. If you are interested in this aspect, be sure to visit the Nordic Heritage Museum in NW 67th Street at 30th Avenue NW.

The most exciting attraction in Ballard, however, is the Hiram Chittenden Locks. To get there from our nominal route termination point, head a few blocks west on NW Market Street to where NW 54ᵗʰ Street peels off to the left. In the latter street, you find the entrance to the Locks. The visitor center is very helpful, providing free maps and brochures.

The Lake Washington Ship Canal was an important strategic development, opening up ocean-going ship access to the timber and coal resources inland from Lake Washington. The canal was completed in 1917, and continues to be in heavy use today. It is an interesting project in that it links the fresh-water Lake Washington system to the salt-water Puget Sound. The Chittenden Locks form a fundamental part of the canal, providing basic separation between the fresh and salt water bodies of water, plus the means for maintaining the desired lake water level independent of ocean tides.

Integrated with the locks is a sophisticated fish ladder system. The fish ladder makes it possible for anadromous fish, such as salmon, to live at sea but migrate to the fresh water lakes and streams to spawn. The fish ladder is set up to allow for spectator viewing of the fish as they travel through it or rest in it. It is not to be missed!

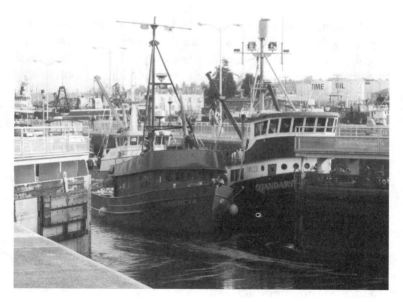

**A Chittenden Locks Gate Opens to Allow Passage of Ocean-Bound Shipping**

In addition, there are attractive Botanical Gardens at the Locks site. Entrance to all these facilities, maintained and operated by the U.S. Army Corps of Engineers, is free.

If you are hungry now, the Lockspot Café near the entrance to the locks on NW 54th Street is a popular place.

There is frequent bus service back downtown, seven days a week, via either the number 17 or number 18 bus. Catch either bus in NW Market Street at Ballard Avenue NW.

# Other Ideas

Since our four routes described above go close to touching each other at a couple of points, there is clearly an opportunity to devise routes that link up pieces of these routes. Here are some possibilities:

- At the Chittenden Locks at the end of our route to Ballard, you can cross the canal and enter Commodore Park, which is a short walk from Discovery Park where our first route starts. Various possibilities present themselves here.

- After doing a loop of Green Lake, there are at least two practical ways of linking up with the Burke-Gilman trail. The first involves going to Fremont as we have described, and then picking up the Burke-Gilman Trail (which itself goes through Fremont) in either direction. The second possibility is to exit Green Lake at its eastern end and follow Northeast Ravenna Boulevard to Ravenna Park. The trail through Ravenna Park takes you to 25th Avenue NE, near to the Burke-Gilman Trail in the University District.

- The start of our third route in Montlake is just across the canal from the University of Washington, and not far from the Burke-Gilman trail where it traverses the campus. It is possible to link up the routes here.

Also, our routes did not fully traverse two of the trails. The first is the **Burke-Gilman Trail**, which extends northeastwards, well beyond what we covered in our fourth route. Also, the trail southward along the **Lake Washington shore** extends well beyond the coverage in our third route. The main reason we did not pursue those extensions is the absence of suitable public transit to or from the endpoints, but if you have other ways around that problem then both options are appealing.

Another route we enjoyed was the two-mile route along **Alki Beach**, where the Denny party first landed in 1851. This is a very attractive on-foot route, with a good beach, scenic views of downtown Seattle, and a range of casual restaurants. However, it is quite short and is not easy to access via public transit. If you have the opportunity to drive there, do so. You will enjoy the run along the beach and back.

\* \* \* \*

Seattle is a very enjoyable city to visit and it offers some exceptional opportunities for on-foot exercise and exploration. If you ever have the chance to get out on-foot here, do not fail to grasp that opportunity and have a ton of fun!

# 13

# City by the Bay

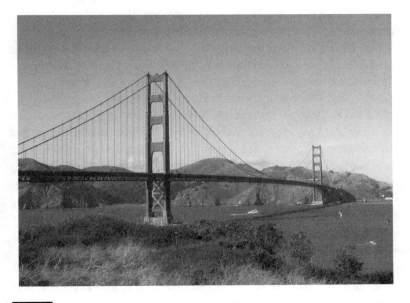

There is something very special about San Francisco. Nola and I have visited this city many times over the past 30 years, and every time has been memorable. In addition to its scenic beauty and dream climate, San Francisco has a magical way of springing pleasant surprises on you at every turn.

In fact, San Francisco helped inspire this book. It is one place where completing an eight-mile run has always proved a mindless and highly rewarding exercise for us—in particular, the outstanding route from Fisherman's Wharf to Sausalito, which we have run many times.

There are two things that make San Francisco particularly appealing for outdoor on-foot activities. The first is the set of scenic routes resulting from the city's location on the Pacific Ocean and the enormous natural harbor and associated waterways that constitute "The Bay." The second is the weather. The monthly average maximum temperature lies between 56 and 70 degrees Fahrenheit year-round, and the monthly average minimum lies between 46 and 56. It is very unlikely you will encounter a temperature outside our preferred range of 40-to-80 degrees. Furthermore, San Francisco's rainy days average a mere 67 days annually. The only weather condition that might discourage on-footers is fog. Fog is a standard part of the San Francisco scene, but it need not inhibit your outdoor venturing. In fact, fog can add a sense of mystery and excitement to your expeditions and, most days, it disappears sometime in the middle of the day anyway.

One of our most memorable runs across the Golden Gate Bridge was in November 2001, on the weekend following California Governor Gray Davis' disclosure of FBI warnings of possible terrorist attacks on U.S. west coast suspension bridges. Davis said National Guard, California Highway Patrol, and U.S. Coast Guard members would be patrolling the Golden Gate and other key bridges. This was in that unforgettable period of grave security fears, less than two months after the 9/11 attacks. Despite this dramatic backdrop, we headed out on our run. It turned out to be one of those days when the Golden Gate was entirely blanketed in fog. Traversing the Golden Gate on foot in fog is an eerie experience at the best of times—the absence of visibility and the bridge's foghorns create an atmosphere that Alfred Hitchcock would have aspired to create.

At the approach onto the bridge's walkway we debated whether to proceed. There were no other pedestrians to be seen. (If the National Guard or California Highway Patrol were there, they sure hid themselves well.) We bravely (or foolishly, we were wondering) decided to push on. The crossing was exceedingly eerie. An unmarked helicopter that could be heard in the fog and mysteriously appeared on occasion did nothing but raise our fears. (For all we could tell, it was the bad guys.) We encountered almost no other foot traffic on the bridge that day. However, as we approached the northern end of the bridge (with a definite feeling of relief), the fog miraculously cleared, as it so often does. We proceeded on to finish one of the most pleasant executions of our favorite running route in gorgeous sunshine. We also seized the occasion to agree that we would never let terrorist fears get in the way of our fun-on-foot agenda in the future.

* * * *

Californians, in general, consider their automobiles to be fundamental extensions of their human bodies. In central San Francisco, this attitude breaks down a little, thanks to a quite good taxi system, a comprehensive public transit network, and outrageous parking costs. The public transit system includes a bewildering mix of buses, streetcars, over/underground light rail (the Muni Metro), regional underground (BART), extra-regional rail (Caltrain), and, of course the famous cable cars. Travel by foot is also considered a quite socially acceptable activity here. As a piece of friendly advice, if you are ever in a hurry and are considering taking a cable car in tourist season, you will likely find the on-foot approach a faster alternative.

This city's violent crime index is 7.4 (offenses per 1,000 residents in 2003)—comparatively respectable for a U.S. city.

San Francisco's best running/jogging/walking routes revolve around the bay shore, the ocean shore, and Golden Gate Park. We see Fisherman's Wharf as a logical center for starting or ending on-foot outings. It has several hotels, much action, and many sights to see. It can also be easily reached on-foot or by public transit from all parts of downtown. If you decide to drive to Fisherman's Wharf, just one word of caution: Parking costs around there verge on mind boggling.

We shall feature three routes, all of which meet our selection criteria outstandingly. Two of them start at Fisherman's Wharf.

| Route | Distance |
|---|---|
| 1. Fisherman's Wharf to Sausalito | 8.0 miles |
| 2. Fisherman's Wharf to Ocean Beach | 10.0 miles |
| 3. Golden Gate Park | 8.0 miles |

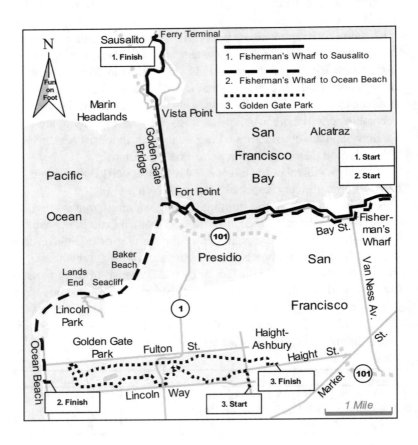

**San Francisco Routes**

# Fisherman's Wharf to Sausalito

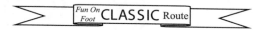

| Distance | 8.0 miles |
| --- | --- |
| Comfort | Excellent running or walking conditions on mainly dedicated pedestrian paths for the first six miles, but some need to follow lightly trafficked roads the last two miles. There are a few short grades. Expect many on-foot exercisers and others for the first six miles, with fewer the last two miles. Some parts are not suitable for inline skating. |
| Attractions | Spectacular views of the San Francisco Bay from the bayside trail, the Golden Gate Bridge, and Vista Point. Views of downtown from the latter two. The ferry ride back is also scenic and exhilarating, usually passing close to Alcatraz. |
| Convenience | Start at Fisherman's Wharf, which can be easily reached on-foot or by bus, streetcar, or cable car from anywhere downtown. End at Sausalito, from where there is a convenient ferry ride back to Fisherman's Wharf or Market Street. |
| Destination | Sausalito, an attractive bayside town with many small shops and several good eating and drinking establishments. Take the ferry back across the bay to San Francisco. |

Our first featured route is the one we mentioned earlier—Fisherman's Wharf to Sausalito via the Golden Gate Bridge, returning via the Sausalito Ferry. While the first part of this route—along the Bay to the bridge—is well known and popular, the continuation to Sausalito is less utilized by runners and walkers. Most pedestrians tend to go onto the bridge then turn back. Many cyclists and a few pedestrians continue on to Sausalito.

Start out from Fisherman's Wharf heading west along the Bay. One of the nice things about on-foot exercise in San Francisco is that you generally do not have to carry much. It is unlikely you will need much clothing for warmth purposes, although it is a good idea to take some sort of shower-proof windbreaker on this route, to help combat the possible effects of fog, wind, and sea spray.

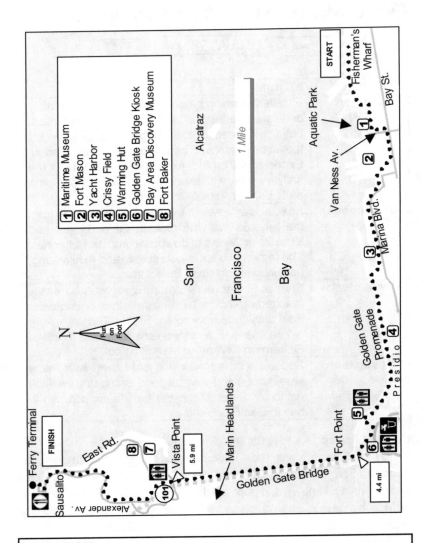

**VARIATION**

Instead of starting at Fisherman's Wharf, you can start in the financial district at Market Street and Embarcadero, and run or walk an additional 1.8 miles to Fisherman's Wharf along the Bay. When returning from Sausalito, take the Golden Gate Ferry that goes to the financial district, rather than the Blue and Gold Ferry to Fisherman's Wharf.

One of the first landmarks you pass is Aquatic Park and its fleet of national historic landmark vessels. You then come to Fort Mason, former military base but now home to various museums and cultural activities. You can work your way through the Fort property but that involves some twisting, turning, and climbing. If you are more interested in getting your on-foot exercise under way than in sightseeing the Fort, we suggest you bypass the Fort by taking Bay Street then cutting back to the bay shore through the grassy area southwest of the Fort. This brings you to Marina Boulevard and a very pleasant pedestrian environment not far from the water. Traversing the Marina area you pass the Yacht Harbor and have the opportunity to ogle some of the finest sailing craft around.

You now enter the Presidio area which extends to the bridge and beyond to the south. The Presidio was founded by the Bay area's first colonizing party in 1776. It was used as a military base by Spain, Mexico, and the United States until the Department of Defense released it to the National Park Service in 1994. The U.S. military used the Presidio as a logistical base for the country's major conflicts since the Spanish-American War in 1898. It is now being transformed into a peaceful national park in which people play, live, and work—and yes, with plenty of paths for joggers and walkers.

You pass along East Beach then through Crissy Field, a pioneering military airfield in the 1920s and now national parkland. There are a couple of different paths through here but the most pleasant is generally that closest to the water, the Golden Gate Promenade.

You come to Torpedo Wharf, where there is a warming hut and public restrooms. If you continued along the water here you would get to Fort Point. However, to get onto the bridge, you need to start climbing here. There is a footpath up the incline to the upper road, which takes you to the Golden Gate Bridge viewing area and kiosk. Unless you are very fit, you may find the climb too much for running, so take a break from running for this little stretch. There are restrooms near the kiosk and you can also buy bottled water and snacks here.

Follow the path from the kiosk up towards the main roadway. This brings you to the bridge walkway. Use the walkway on the eastern side of the bridge. This walkway is conveniently reserved for pedestrian traffic on weekends; cyclists must use the western walkway. The walkways are closed at night.

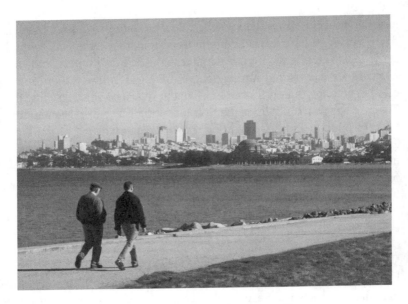

The Golden Gate Promenade

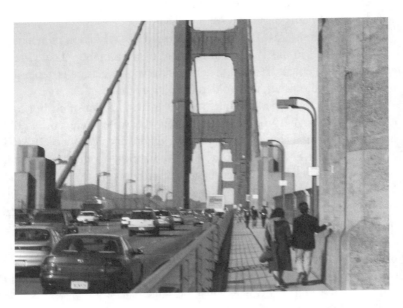

Golden Gate Bridge Eastern Walkway

Construction of the Golden Gate Bridge began in 1933. The bridge opened in 1937, at that time the world's longest suspension bridge (not surpassed until the opening of New York's Verrazano-Narrows Bridge in 1964). The towers are 4,200 feet apart and 746 feet high above the water.

The cost of construction was $35 million. In 2004 dollars, I calculated that at $455 million.[1] The Golden Gate Bridge website estimates the cost to build the bridge in 2003 at $1.2 billion.[2] (The difference between these two figures is attributed to such factors as environmental reviews and costs of materials and labor.)

Compare either of those figures with the $14 billion cost of Boston's Big Dig. The construction of the Golden Gate Bridge, from scratch, cost 3%-to-9% of a project to relocate a few miles of highway from a poorly designed 40-year old elevated expressway to an underground tunnel below it! And the Golden Gate, without significant change, continues to serve its community admirably in a critically essential role, 70 years after it was built. Even today, you could build ten Golden Gates for what the Big Dig cost.

The American Society of Civil Engineers classified the Golden Gate as one of the modern Seven Wonders of the World. That recognition is clearly well deserved—right up to today.

The bridge crossing is spectacular. Not only do you get to observe at close quarters the bridge's fascinating construction (the whole structure hangs off a couple of three-feet diameter cables that you can touch), but you also get an outstanding view of San Francisco Bay. The view typically includes recreational and racing sailing craft, commercial shipping, naval vessels, Alcatraz, and the San Francisco city skyline.

As you exit the bridge walkway at the northern end and enter Marin County, you come to Vista Point. This is where the unfit of our community drive to and park with the hope of experiencing the view we have just had on the bridge. They get a pretty good view here but it does not compare with the real thing. There are restrooms at Vista Point.

There are a couple of possible routes from here to Sausalito. The most direct one is 2.1 miles via Alexander Avenue. As you leave the

1        Calculated using the Federal Reserve's Consumer Price Index calculator.
2        The Golden Gate Bridge website http://www.goldengatebridge.org is the source of most of the bridge facts we state here.

Vista Point area, follow the road northbound that looks like it is going to put you onto highway 101, but keep to the paved path to the far right. This path leads you onto the Alexander Avenue highway exit.

As a word of caution, there is no bicycle path and a very rudimentary pedestrian path along Alexander Avenue. You need to be prepared to travel virtually on the edge of the road pavement. However, Alexander Avenue has quite light vehicular traffic while having its fair share of cyclist traffic. As a pedestrian, keep to the extreme right, and take extra care.

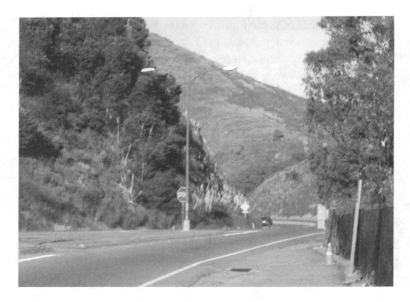

**Alexander Avenue**

Pedestrians on this route around April-May are treated to a special bonus. The sides of Alexander Avenue and adjacent terrain are endowed with an exceptional wildflower display and pedestrians experience this at first hand. Marin County is famous for the continuing presence of the wildflowers that once graced all of California.[3]

As you progress up Alexander Avenue, the pedestrian space starts to become extremely narrow and questionable as you approach the highest cutting. However, do not despair since, as soon as you get through that

---

3        There is an excellent document describing the different wildflowers at: http://www.nps.gov/gpga/maps/bulletins/sb-wildflwrs.pdf.

cutting, you enter a new world of wider and safer pedestrian space. It is also now downhill all the way, with gorgeous views of the Sausalito and Tiburon parts of the bay. Furthermore, if you have been troubled by wind, fog, damp, or cold during the run over the bridge, as you approach Sausalito you enter a new climate zone. This area is well protected from the weather forces of the Pacific Ocean by the mountains of the Marin peninsula, and temperatures and other weather phenomena are often much more friendly than other parts of the Bay.

---

**VARIATION**

An alternative to following the edge of Alexander Avenue is to take the lower-level Bay Trail, which goes past the old Coast Guard station, Fort Baker, and the San Francisco Bay Children's Discovery center. This route has a few more things to see but will take somewhat longer. To get to it, head firstly towards Alexander Avenue, but then take the road tunnel under Route 101 to its western side. Bear left and follow the winding path down almost to the water level. You here intersect a pedestrian/bicycle path that takes you eastward under the bridge approach. It then continues on around the coastline, following East Road and eventually linking you up again with Alexander Avenue quite close to Sausalito.

---

As you continue on Alexander Avenue down into Sausalito, keep bearing right and you end up on the Sausalito foreshore. You are probably ready to wind up your exercise activity on reaching this very pleasant town. In Sausalito, you can spend as much time as you want exploring the multitude of local shops (antiques, general tourist fare, and sundry other offerings) and other establishments. Plan on catching the ferry back to the city at your leisure.

There are various eating and drinking establishments. If you like the idea of a good mid-market pub-restaurant, willing to accommodate damp and disheveled on-footers, we can personally recommend the Water Street Grille. It has great food, staff, and atmosphere, with a patio on the Bay shore where you can contemplate San Francisco's skyline. If you like seafood and do not mind paying a little more, Scoma's (which is on the water's edge nearby) is another recommendation. When we were last in Sausalito, weekend brunch was offered at both establishments.

---

After eating, drinking, and shopping to your heart's content, you can catch either the Blue and Gold ferry back to Fisherman's Wharf or the Golden Gate Ferry to Embarcadero and Market Street. The ferry schedules vary year-round so it is a good idea to pick up a schedule from a hotel concierge or website before you start out. The ferries typically run every one-to-two hours. You do not need a ticket in advance—buy it on board. The ticket price is reasonable and the ride typically takes around 30 minutes.

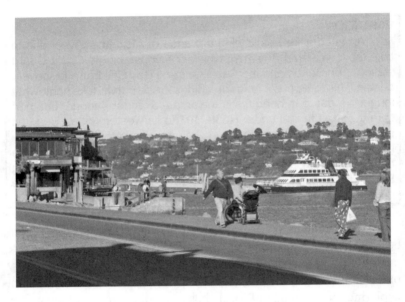

**The Sausalito Foreshore, Water Street Grille on the left and the Ferry Dock at Rear**

The ferry ride is also mighty spectacular. You get to see the Bay's sea craft at close hand, along with scenic views of the Golden Gate, Alcatraz, and the approaching San Francisco skyline. The ferries have restrooms. As you disembark at Fisherman's Wharf or Market Street, you are most likely feeling pretty good about the whole experience you have just had...

\* \* \* \*

The route we just described has an interesting characteristic. After completing around three quarters of the route, you effectively reach a point of no return. Once you get towards the northern end of the bridge, there is virtually no point turning back. The effort you faced would be as much as if you continue on to Sausalito and it would be far less interesting. We find this characteristic of certain running routes very helpful since it eliminates the temptation to cut the run short, just because some of those pesky muscles or joints are starting to ache.

# Fisherman's Wharf to Ocean Beach

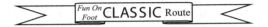

NOTE:  You need to refer to our Fisherman's Wharf to Sausalito route description for directions for the first part of this route.

| Distance | 10.0 miles |
|---|---|
| Comfort | Excellent running or walking conditions on mainly dedicated pedestrian paths for the first 4.4 miles. After that, the terrain becomes more demanding, with some grades and less well manicured trails. However, the paths are generally dedicated to pedestrians, with the occasional need to follow a street sidewalk.  Expect many on-foot exercisers throughout the route.   Not suitable for inline skating. |
| Attractions | A scenic bonanza!  Spectacular views of the San Francisco Bay from the bayside trail, then scenic overlooks of the rugged Pacific Ocean shore from the oceanside trail.  Also pass the classy residential area of Seacliff, famous Lands End, sandy Ocean Beach, and the western end of Golden Gate Park. |
| Convenience | Start at Fisherman's Wharf, which can be easily reached on-foot or by bus, streetcar, or cable car from anywhere downtown.  End at Ocean Beach, roughly six miles west of downtown.  There is public transit back downtown via the Muni Metro N-line at its Judah Street terminus, or via various Muni Bus routes. |
| Destination | Ocean Beach, on the western edge of Golden Gate Park.  There is an attractive beach environment and an excellent wind-down restaurant here—the Beach Chalet. If you want to continue into Golden Gate Park, there are various sights nearby. |

Our second San Francisco route shares some common ground with the first route, but has its own special features.  The first 4.4 miles of the route are the same as the first route—from Fisherman's Wharf to the Golden Gate Bridge kiosk.  However, from the kiosk we follow

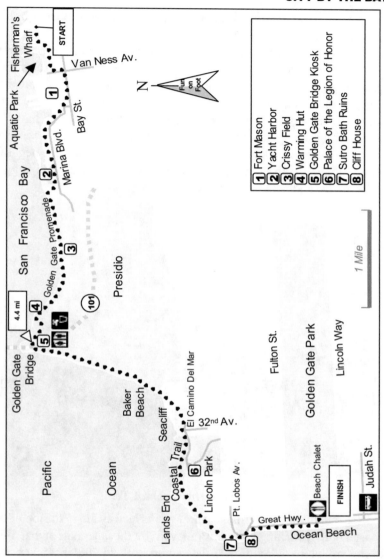

START

Fisherman's
Wharf

Van Ness Av.

Aquatic Park

1

San Francisco Bay

2

Marina Blvd.

Bay St.

N

Fun
on
Foot

Golden Gate Promenade

3

Presidio

101

4.4 mi

4

5

Golden Gate Bridge

Pacific

Ocean

Baker Beach

Seacliff

Lands End

Coastal Trail

El Camino Del Mar

32nd Av.

6

Lincoln Park

Pt. Lobos Av.

7  8

Great Hwy.

Ocean Beach

Fulton St.

Golden Gate Park

Lincoln Way

Beach Chalet

FINISH

Judah St.

1 Mile

1 Fort Mason
2 Yacht Harbor
3 Crissy Field
4 Warming Hut
5 Golden Gate Bridge Kiosk
6 Palace of the Legion of Honor
7 Sutro Bath Ruins
8 Cliff House

the ocean coast southward this time, continuing as far as Golden Gate Park.

From the kiosk you need to cross Route 101 to pick up the Bay Ridge Coastal Trail. The easiest way is a bicycle and pedestrian underpass under the approach to the bridge. This takes you directly to the start of the ocean trail. Alternatively, if you cannot find that underpass, you can use the road underpass under the toll plaza then bear right to link up with the trail.

Let us warn you at the outset about some aspects of the Coastal Trail. First, in some parts, it would probably be more accurately classified as a hiking trail than a running trail. While much of it is runnable, it gets a little steep in spots and a little rough underfoot. Second, the weather conditions here can be much wilder than inside the bay. Be prepared for stronger winds, together with sea spray and heavier fog than you experience bayside. However, the flipside of these negative characteristics is the outstanding ocean view, complete with rugged cliffs, rocks, and pounding waves.

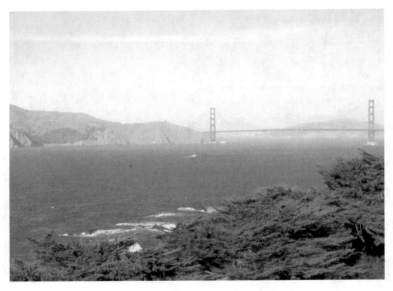

**Vista from the Coastal Trail**

For roughly the first mile, the trail works its way along the top of the coastal bluffs, tracking Lincoln Boulevard for the latter part of that mile. If you are interested in turn-of-the-century (19th to 20th, that is) coastal defense batteries, you will pass several of them at first hand. When you get to the point where the bluffs become lower and you are overlooking Baker Beach, watch for and follow the path that takes you down to the beach-level battery. Continue at the beach level for about 0.3 mile until you run out of path at that level and are forced to start climbing again, this time into what is clearly a more residential precinct.

The area you are about to enter is known as Seacliff. It is impressive in its own right, mainly for the class of the residences perched on the cliffs here. Keep heading south until you encounter the street called El Camino Del Mar, which you then follow westward to Lincoln Park.

There are various ways to negotiate Lincoln Park from its northeastern corner to its southwestern corner. The most popular is the Coastal Trail, which you can enter from El Camino del Mar just after 32nd Avenue, and follow high above the cliffs through the park. There are a few grades to deal with, but it does offer very scenic views. For something even more daring and spectacular, explore the complex network of cliff paths, but be careful! If you are not in a hurry, consider making a side trip down the trail to Lands End beach. There is also a more conservative route through the park: Follow El Camino del Mar to the Palace of the Legion of Honor (where Rodin's bronze *Thinker* contemplates; just like in Philadelphia, New York, and a few other places); then continue straight ahead on Upper Legion Trail, which follows the coast above the Coastal Trail.

Whichever route you choose, you end up at the southwestern corner of Lincoln Park. On the coast here are the ruins of the Sutro Baths—a turn-of-the-century three-plus acre water park. It could accommodate 10,000 guests and included a 3,700-seat amphitheatre, restaurants seating 1,000, and impressive art galleries. The venture was never an outstanding commercial success and a fire in 1966 sealed its fate.

South of those ruins is the Cliff House, another famous establishment, with a history extending back to 1863. However, the Cliff House is still alive and well today. It has a restaurant and bar. The food and atmosphere are excellent, but a little on the up-market side. A weekend brunch is offered.

We suggest you continue a further 0.8 mile south along Ocean Beach. This is an enormous, beautiful, sandy beach but not (so we hear) a particularly safe or pleasant bathing spot. To complete your on-foot route, follow the beach, with the (euphemistically named) Great Highway on your left. Enjoy the exposure to the natural forces of the Pacific Ocean. In due course, the landscape across the road changes from buildings to trees, heralding the start of Golden Gate Park. Cross the road and continue a short way south to the Beach Chalet.

The Beach Chalet is an excellent termination point for this on-foot outing. It has a great view and great food, including breakfast daily and brunch on weekends. It has its own brewpub. It also acts as a gateway to Golden Gate Park, with a Visitor Center right in the building. (See our next route for on-foot ideas in Golden Gate Park.)

Furthermore, the Beach Chalet is moderately convenient to fast public transit back to central San Francisco. Continue on foot southward on Great Highway to Lincoln Way at the southern end of Golden Gate Park, then go a further two streets to Judah Street. Here you can catch the Muni Metro N line, which will take you the full west-to-east breadth of the park and on to downtown. In the downtown area, the rail car travels under Market Street from Van Ness Avenue to Embarcadero. To get back to Fisherman's Wharf you can disembark at Powell Street and take the Powell-Mason cable car or, if the line is too long, walk or hail a taxi. If using the Muni, be aware you need correct change, so carry a few singles and quarters with you.

Nola and I will never forget our first run on this route. The very positive aspects of the route (great scenery, interesting places en route, good pub at the end, etc.) were somewhat dampened by, well… *dampness*. It was not a rainy day but it was a very *damp* day. The atmosphere would probably be classified as fog or mist; certainly humidity was 100%. The combined result from this atmosphere, the ocean spray, and the perspiration from running meant that, regardless of how you dressed, you would end up totally soaked. And we were. We were very glad to reach the Beach Chalet, albeit in somewhat bedraggled condition. However, the warmth, good food, friendly atmosphere, and a few alcoholic pleasures succeeded in restoring our spirits from a one to a nine. Depending on the weather for your outing, you might want to be mentally prepared for a similar situation.

\* \* \* \*

The two instances of "Coastal Trail" we mentioned above are not only nice local foot trails but also part of a much grander State project called the California Coastal Trail (CCT). The plan calls for the eventual construction of a walkable trail extending the entire length of the California coastline. This is a fascinating concept. It is enormously challenging, given the number of authorities and private landowners involved, not to mention the geographical feature challenges. It is real, though, at least at the political level—in 2000 the State legislature declared the CCT an official state trail and President Clinton declared it a Millennium Heritage Trail. Its development continues…

# Golden Gate Park

| Distance | 8.0 miles |
|---|---|
| Comfort | Excellent underfoot conditions. There are many on-foot exercisers, cyclists, and others around in most of the park, but note that it is a large park with some isolated spots. Around the Haight Street park entrance, don't be surprised to encounter several homeless people. There is considerable vehicle traffic but judicious route choice can minimize traffic encounters. Our recommended route is not suitable for inline skating but alternative routes in the park are. |
| Attractions | A large area of green space, with various sights, such as a traversable botanic garden, several attractive lakes, two waterfalls, a Japanese Tea Garden, a Conservatory of Flowers, a field of bison, and two interesting windmills. |
| Convenience | Start and end in the Haight-Ashbury area, roughly three miles west of downtown. It can be conveniently reached from Market Street via the Muni Metro N Line. |
| Destination | Haight-Ashbury, an area with tremendous character. There are several good eating and drinking establishments and numerous shops. |

Golden Gate Park is San Francisco's closest equivalent to New York's Central Park. Golden Gate Park, with 1,017 acres, is a little larger than 843-acre Central Park. Both have similar attractions, including nice landscaping, community activities, and interesting cultural destinations. Golden Gate Park is more vehicle-infested than Central Park (but, after all, this is California). Also, Golden Gate Park is just not so central as Central Park. To get to Golden Gate Park from downtown (three miles or so), no direct on-foot route is particularly attractive, thanks to San Francisco's ubiquitous hills and traffic. However, there is reasonably convenient public transit and, if you make the effort to come here, we think you will definitely appreciate it afterwards.

Golden Gate Park was established in 1870, on a site consisting mainly of sand dunes, somewhat removed from what was then the city of San Francisco. Its main period of development, however, is

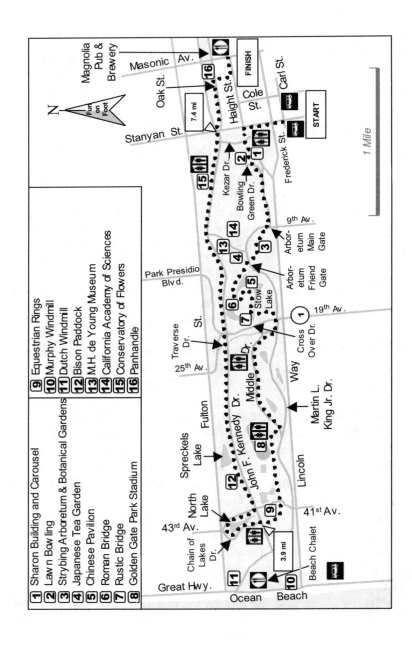

recognized as the 56-year period beginning in 1887 when Scotsman John McLaren was its superintendent. McLaren planted a massive number of trees and plants and successfully converted the formerly arid land to green space. Under McLaren's supervision, the park, essentially as it is today, was developed.

This is a large and complex park. There are many things to see and many different trail choices. We shall lay out one suggested route but we have no doubt you will find ways to vary that route to best suit your own tastes.

One unfortunate aspect is the large amount of motor vehicle traffic in the park. It can, however, be largely avoided—we do our best to do that in the route suggested below.

We start at the southeastern corner of the park. Using public transit you can easily get here from downtown by catching the Muni Metro N line in Market Street to the Stanyan Street stop. Then head north along Stanyan Street, going two short blocks to Haight Street. Enter the park here, picking up the paved pedestrian trail. One of the nice things about entering here is that you can use a pedestrian underpass under busy Kezar Drive and so can keep away from vehicle encounters for quite a while.

Follow the trail westward. Pass Mothers' Meadow, a popular location for children's sporting events. Head directly to the distinctive Sharon Building, passing the children's playground and the carousel on your left. The pedestrian path eventually leads to Bowling Green Drive, after negotiating the lawn bowling club's car park. Take Bowling Green Drive to the left. It connects with Martin Luther King Jr. Drive, the main traffic throughway along the southern side of the park. This road has a good sidewalk and the traffic is tolerable for the short distance you need to follow the road.

Follow MLK Drive to the T-intersection at 9th Avenue where you see the San Francisco County Fair Building dead ahead. Next to that building is what caused us to direct you to this part of the park—the main gate of the Strybing Arboretum and Botanical Gardens. This is an excellent place for on-foot exercisers. Bicycles are not permitted but joggers are welcome and there is no charge. You have a choice of routes through the gardens, emerging at a second gate known variously as the Friend Gate or North Entrance. The 55-acre gardens contain over 7,000 kinds of plants, featuring collections of plants from Asia,

Australia, South Africa, Chile, Mexico, Central America, New Zealand, and, less surprisingly, California. You can pick up a free map at the little bookstore just inside the main entrance and use this to shape your route to see your favorite plant category.

The Friend Gate brings you out again on MLK Drive. Cross that road and pick up the little trail that takes you northwesterly. On your right is the Japanese Tea Garden—originally the Japanese Village of the 1894 Midwinter International Exposition. The trail leads you to the eastern end of Stow Lake, one of the nicest, and more hidden, parts of the park. Stow Lake was established in the 1890's as a reservoir, with attractive landscaping and paths to serve its visitors. Until the 1906 earthquake took its toll, the elaborate Sweeny Observatory graced Strawberry Hill, the 400-foot natural hill on the island in the middle of the lake.

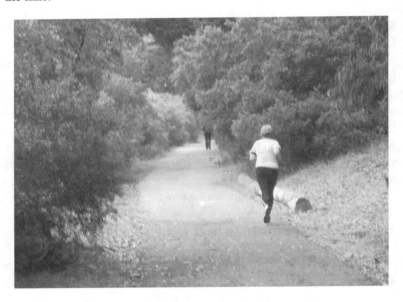

**A Pedestrian Trail in Golden Gate Park**

There are various on-foot options through the Stow Lake area. Take any route that will get you to the southwestern corner of the lake. One option is to follow the northern edge of the lake anticlockwise to the Roman Bridge, and cross that bridge to Strawberry Hill Island. Then take the dirt path clockwise around the edge of the island past the

Chinese Pavilion to the Rustic Bridge. The Chinese Pavilion was a gift from the City of Taipei in 1981. The Rustic Bridge, or Stone Bridge, served the Sweeny Observatory while it sat atop Strawberry Hill.

From the Rustic Bridge or southwestern corner of the lake, work your way south back to MLK Drive. Follow MLK Drive west to the busy intersection with Cross Over Drive, the north-south traffic artery that dissects the park. There is a pedestrian crossing light here.

After negotiating this intersection, there are some new ways to escape road traffic and get closer to nature. Go straight then take the first road to the right, Traverse Drive. After a short distance there is a road off to the left, called Middle Drive. This road is closed to through traffic and sometimes all traffic. This is a nice route to take as an on-foot exerciser, being quiet and devoid of enemy number one.

Middle Drive eventually brings you to the southern entrance to what is variously called the Golden Gate Park Stadium or the Polo Field.

From this point, we suggest you negotiate the small parking area and pick up the paved bicycle/pedestrian trail heading westward. This trail takes you to the western boundary of the park, without requiring you to follow trafficked roads. For our nominal route, we do not go as far as the park's western boundary. Rather we suggest heading north after the Bercut Equitation Ring, to get to the northern side of the park.

---

**VARIATION**

If you are interested in windmills, keep heading westward to the Murphy Windmill (1905) near the southwestern corner of the park, then follow the path northward to the Beach Chalet and, after that, the Dutch Windmill (1902). Then work eastward again to North Lake to pick up our nominal route. This diversion adds roughly one mile to the route.

---

Heading northward from the equestrian rings, you should encounter JFK Drive near the restrooms at the corner of Chain of Lakes Drive West, a road that is now permanently closed to traffic. This is the 3.9-mile point of our route—roughly halfway.

You have an opportunity here to escape from road traffic for a little while longer by following Chain of Lakes Drive West northward, around North Lake. At the northern end of that lake, you meet road traffic again on Chain of Lakes Drive East, but there is a nice pedestrian and bicycle trail on the lakeshore. After almost circumnavigating North Lake, you get back to JFK Drive.

---

**VARIATION**

You can shorten the route by roughly a half-mile by skipping the circumnavigation of North Lake and simply following JFK Drive eastward from the restrooms.

---

JFK Drive is the main road traversing the park east-to-west near its northern edge. There is considerable road traffic and also a lot of pedestrian traffic. The good news is that bicycles are required to use the road, and there is a paved pedestrian trail following the road for most of its length. Use this trail to get back to the eastern edge of the park.

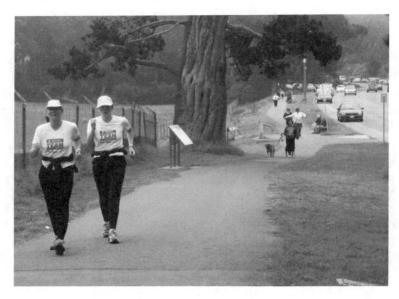

**No Bicycles or Skating Allowed—The Popular John F. Kennedy Drive Pedestrian Side-Trail**

There are a few interesting spectacles en route. The first, not far past Chain of Lakes Drive East, is a paddock of bison on the left. That is quite amazing, really, for a park in the middle of San Francisco. Beyond that, you encounter Spreckels Lake, where miniature power and sail boat enthusiasts play and entertain the passers-by. After that, you pass the Rose Garden on the left. Then you come to the M.H. de Young Museum, which has been an integral and cherished part of Golden Gate Park for over a hundred years. This museum houses a permanent collection of American art from the 17$^{th}$ through 20$^{th}$ centuries, plus art of Africa, Oceania, and the native Americas.

Continue along JFK Drive. You pass, on your left, the Conservatory of Flowers. This Victorian greenhouse is the oldest building in Golden Gate Park, having provided a tropical environment for flower displays since 1879.

Keep following JFK Drive to its end at Stanyan Street. Cross Stanyan Street at the pedestrian crossing and enter the park's panhandle. There is a pedestrian-only trail on the southern side of the panhandle near Oak Street. The main action is two short blocks south of Oak on Haight Street. We shall leave it to you to decide where to leave the panhandle and head south to Haight.

The Haight-Ashbury area is famous as the center of the hippie culture of the 1960s. Today, there is not much evidence of that era left. This is largely a commercial tourist area, with the occasional offbeat twist.

There are many cafés, restaurants, and bars in Haight Street or the side streets. We like the Magnolia Pub and Brewery at Masonic and Haight. It is full of character and has an outstanding range of its own brews and quite reasonable food. On Saturdays and Sundays a comprehensive brunch menu is offered—I much enjoyed my crab cake benedict along with a local brew.

To get from this area back to downtown you have various choices. You might choose to travel on-foot eastward on Haight through the Lower Haight district (more of a nightlife area), and pick up bus transport at various places should you need it. The easier approach, though, is to head south to Cole and Carl Streets to catch the Muni N Line back to Market Street downtown.

# Other Ideas

Our first two routes used the **bayside trail** from Fisherman's Wharf westward to the Golden Gate Bridge. The trail also continues roughly three miles eastward from Fisherman's Wharf as well. It follows Embarcadero through downtown, under the San Francisco-Oakland

Bay Bridge, and as far as the ballpark (home of the Giants) at King Street. You are treated to excellent views of the San Francisco Bay and the city throughout.

Our second route took you to Ocean Beach at Golden Gate Park. The **Ocean Beach trail** continues south from Golden Gate Park, along the ocean shore to the San Francisco Zoo.

Our first route took you across the Golden Gate Bridge to Marin County and Sausalito. Westward from the northern end of the bridge are the **Marin Headlands**. There are many trails through that area, and spectacular views. However, the climbs are quite steep so bear that in mind.

* * * *

San Francisco is the classic city for finding your own comfort zone— satisfying your own cultural, eating, entertainment, and socializing preferences. Nola and I have never failed to find our level here, and we have no doubt you can too.

Despite the automobiles, this really is an on-foot-friendly city. There are some outstanding on-foot experiences awaiting you if you venture out. We hope our route descriptions help you put together a truly memorable on-foot adventure while in the City by the Bay.

# 14

# City of Angels

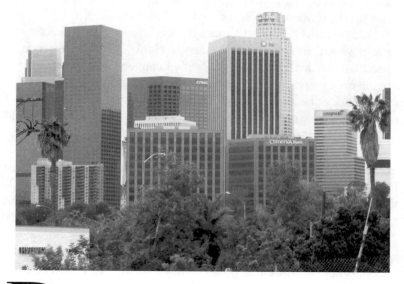

**D**oes anyone enjoy spending time out on foot in Los Angeles, the number one city for automobile dependence? That seemed a good question to us. Given LA's size, we figured we absolutely must give this city the same sort of analysis we gave the other major cities.

We quickly concluded that Los Angeles is not without its hazards for the on-foot exerciser. Firstly, neighborhood gangs and recreational runners do not make a good mix. LA has a less than perfect reputation in that respect, especially its east side and south-central area. LA's violent crime index is 12.7 (crimes per 1,000 residents in 2003), higher than average but far from the worst U.S. city. Being prudent, we decided to limit our route consideration to the slab of LA from downtown westward to the coast. This area, which generally has a good reputation, also has much to offer in the way of beaches, parks, and hills—features that tend to go along with good on-foot exercise routes.

The automobile is probably a bigger hazard than street security. LA pedestrians and automobiles have a unique relationship, which comes to the forefront at the traffic signal. LA is the only city in the United States where all pedestrians religiously follow the directions of the pedestrian crossing lights. If you are on-foot, wait at each traffic light until the little white man flashes walk. Do not contemplate doing otherwise. If there is no pedestrian crossing with a little white man, then find one. Then find the button to press (often a challenge in itself).

There are two very good reasons for this behavior. First, LA drivers have a vision affliction that selectively blanks out the existence of pedestrians on the retina's image, so if you are on a road when a car is driving on it you are more than likely already dead. Second, there is a definite risk of being booked by LA police for jaywalking. The LAPD really hate removing human road kill and therefore aggressively uphold all laws applying to pedestrians.

Let us now move on to the number one positive aspect of on-foot exercise in LA—the weather. LA's average maximum temperature lies between our desired 40-to-80 degrees Fahrenheit range most of the year, just sneaking above 80 in July, August, and September. The average minimum is above 40 year-round. On average, there are only 35 rainy days per year, so precipitation is unlikely to cause you a major problem.

LA is not famous for its public transit system. Nevertheless, as in all cities we cover, we wanted to find on-foot routes that do not depend upon use of an automobile for their execution. This was an interesting learning experience.

We had some difficulty finding out about the bus system, in particular. We asked various people, from our hotel concierge to the assistants in the local bookstore and the city information kiosk. They all tried to help but could not really give convincing or accurate answers. We eventually worked out why. *None of these people had ever actually used a bus in their lives.*

We tried in vain to acquire a printed regional transit map. If one does exist, we could not find the right person to point us to it.

We fell back to the Internet, where some helpful websites indeed exist.[1] Then we explored the public transit services for ourselves. The results surprised us. There are actually some excellent public transit services in LA—fast, frequent, and clean, with courteous and helpful staff. We encountered no nasty surprises. Clearly the LA public transit system is somewhat underrated.

We found two particularly impressive public transit services for the area in which we were researching on-foot routes. The first is the Red Line Metro train, which runs from downtown westward to the mid-Wilshire area, Hollywood, and the San Fernando Valley. This modern subway system is the cleanest and smoothest you will encounter anywhere in the world. The second impressive service is the bus network, including Big Blue and Metro buses, that serves the coastal communities west of downtown. The network includes the Big Blue Bus Line 10 and the Metro Rapid 720 express services, which move people quite quickly and frequently between Santa Monica and downtown. LA indeed has a public transit system of above average quality.

After much research, we decided to feature three on-foot routes in this chapter. They have differing characteristics and therefore offer you a lot of variety. We shall also discuss other possibilities at the end.

| Route | Distance |
|---|---|
| 1.  Santa Monica to Marina Del Rey | 5.7 miles |
| 2.  Hollywood Hills | 7.5 miles |
| 3.  UCLA to Santa Monica | 7.3 miles |

---

1        Especially http://www.mta.net and http://www.bigbluebus.com.

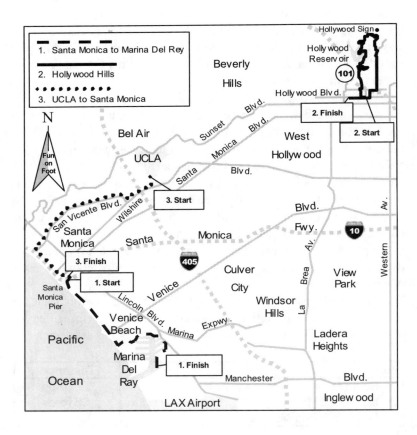

**Los Angeles Routes**

# Santa Monica to Marina Del Rey

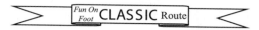

| Distance | 5.7 miles |
|---|---|
| **Comfort** | Excellent running or walking conditions on dedicated pedestrian or pedestrian/bicycle paths. The entire route is flat. Expect many people around, including a good number of other on-foot exercisers. The beach is patrolled. OK for inline skating. |
| **Attractions** | Beautiful sandy beaches with many people enjoying them. A busy street market environment on weekends in the Venice Beach area. See classy sailing and motorized sea craft at the marina. |
| **Convenience** | Start in Santa Monica, which can be easily reached from downtown Los Angeles via express Big Blue Bus Line 10 or Metro Rapid 720 bus. End at Marina Del Rey, where there is regular Big Blue Bus Line 3 service back to Santa Monica. This route also works fine in the opposite direction. |
| **Destination** | Fisherman's Village at Marina Del Rey, an attractive wind-down spot with eating and drinking establishments overlooking the marina channel. If you do this route the opposite way, you end in Santa Monica, with abundant restaurant, bar, and shopping selections. Either way, there is convenient public transit back to the start point via the Big Blue Bus. |

Los Angeles has one outstanding feature for the outdoor-inclined—the string of beautiful Pacific Ocean beaches stretching virtually the entire western perimeter of the metropolis.

We chose to cover a piece of this beachfront that fits all of our criteria particularly well. This is the stretch between the lovely seaside city of Santa Monica and the classy marina district of Marina Del Rey. Both end points have a choice of hotel accommodations so, if you are a visitor to the region, you might well find yourself staying near one end or the other.

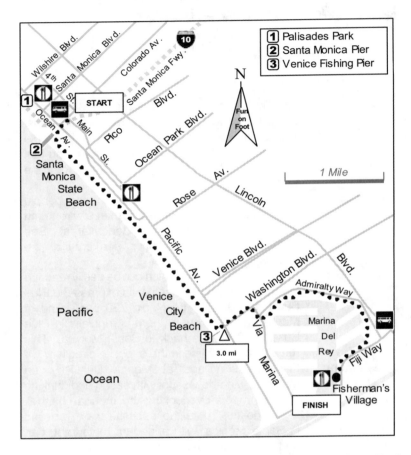

You can execute this route equally well in either direction. Both ends form excellent destination points and there is a good public transit connection between the end-points. We arbitrarily chose to describe the route starting from Santa Monica. Since this route has more than adequate restrooms and water sources along the way, the map does not show those.

You can start out from anywhere in Santa Monica. Just head west toward the coast, pick up the seaside pedestrian or bicycle path, then head south. For distance measurement purposes, we shall assume starting at Colorado Avenue and Main Street, close to the transit, shopping, and restaurant areas of Santa Monica. This point is two short blocks inland from the Santa Monica pier.

The first mile takes you along Santa Monica State Beach. This is as good as on-foot conditions ever get. There are separate pedestrian and bicycle paths. If the former gets a little congested, you can probably get away with jogging on the bicycle path provided you are careful not to unnecessarily impede cyclists. Police patrol the beach and paths regularly. There are snack kiosks and public restrooms.

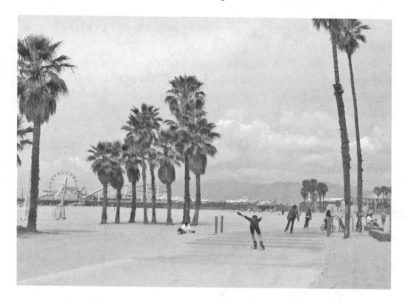

**The Bicycle Path at Santa Monica State Beach**

A block shy of Rose Avenue, you cross the Santa Monica City boundary and enter Venice Beach, part of the City of Los Angeles. You here notice an immediate change in character of the environment.

The on-foot conditions continue to be excellent, with separate bike and pedestrian paths. However, a big difference in the Venice Beach stretch is the existence of numerous commercial activities along the pedestrian paths. There are shops, fast food outlets, pubs, and restaurants. There are sidewalk vendors and a flea-market environment on Friday, Saturday, and Sunday. The attitude is relaxed and pleasant, but be warned that Venice Beach has a reputation as a place to keep away from at night.

Where the bike path ends at Washington Boulevard, turn left and head inland for a short distance to the street on the right called Via

Marina. This street takes you to the largest manmade small boat harbor in the world, accommodating around 7,000 pleasure craft. This is Marina Del Rey.

Where you meet the marina, the street on the left is Admiralty Way. This takes you around the marina to its southern end. However, as a pedestrian, you get a better break than cyclists and motorists. You can, by and large, follow pedestrian paths close to the water and admire the sea craft at close range. You probably want to avoid trekking out onto the marina's piers though.

There is only one significant impediment to pedestrians—the California Yacht Club, which has taken over the waterfront for a chunk of the marina and barred public pedestrian access. Thumbs down to the CYC!

After the CYC and Café Del Rey, a new bike path starts up. This follows Admiralty Way to Fiji Way, and then on to the southern end of the marina. There you find Fisherman's Village, by the Coast Guard Station at the end of the road.

Fisherman's Village is billed in the tourist literature as a model of a New England fishing village. This stretches the imagination somewhat, but it is indeed a pleasant place to end an on-foot outing.

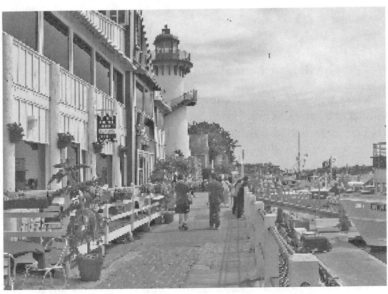

**Fisherman's Village at Marina Del Rey**

If you are ready for food or a drink after your exercise, there are restaurants at Fisherman's Village, most with a good view of the marina channel and its busy sea craft traffic to and from the ocean. Nola and I settled on El Torito Restaurant and Cantina, a franchise of a Californian chain of Mexican restaurant/pubs. Southern California has excellent Mexican food, and we found this place very satisfactory all round.

To get from Fisherman's Village back to Santa Monica via public transit, retrace your steps up Fiji Way past the Admiralty Way intersection to Lincoln Boulevard. Here you can catch the frequent Big Blue Bus back to central Santa Monica.

As noted in this route's introduction, the route works equally well in the opposite direction, especially if you are staying at a hotel around Marina Del Rey. Simply pick up our route near your hotel and head north to Santa Monica.

In Santa Monica, there are many suitable wind-down places. The establishment that impressed us most was Ye Olde King's Head Restaurant and Pub in Santa Monica Boulevard at 2nd Street. This is a better English pub than most of the modern pubs in England. It has an outstanding menu, including traditional English pub fare and also food with flavors more attractive to the American palate. We found a good mix of backgrounds in the clientele here, including British ex-pats, Santa Monica locals, and American visitors to town. This establishment is close to the center of the Third Street Promenade pedestrian and shopping precinct.

Another fine establishment we liked was Finn McCool's Irish Pub at 2700 Main Street, a few blocks southeast of Colorado Avenue, near Ocean Park Boulevard. It is a very traditional Irish pub with a good food selection, a largely Irish staff, and evening entertainment. Its interior was transported in pieces from Ireland.

While in Santa Monica you might choose to check out 100-year-old Santa Monica Pier, a popular destination attracting some three million visitors annually. There are amusement park rides, food and drink outlets, and a generally lively scene. North of the pier is the start of Palisades Park, a pleasant park overlooking the ocean and an excellent place for enjoying the sunsets.

You can catch the Big Blue Bus Line 3 back to Marina Del Rey in 4th Street at Santa Monica Boulevard or, if you are in the Main Street precinct, at Ocean Park and Lincoln Boulevard.

---

# Hollywood Hills

| Distance | 7.5 miles |
| --- | --- |
| Comfort | The first half-mile and last mile are along flat sidewalks of busy streets. There are about two miles on flat vehicle-free trails. The remainder follows lightly trafficked streets through quality residential neighborhoods. There are some significant uphill and downhill grades along the residential streets. Expect other people around on most of the route. Not suitable for inline skating. |
| Attractions | Some spectacular residential areas with classy homes perched on elevated crags and bluffs; the Hollywood Reservoir and its vehicle-free wildlife-rich environs; the famous Hollywood Sign at close range; and Hollywood Boulevard's tourist attractions. |
| Convenience | Start and finish on Hollywood Boulevard, close to Red Line Metro train stations, with fast and comfortable service to and from downtown Los Angeles. |
| Destination | Hollywood Boulevard and its entertainment-world attractions, including the Walk of Fame, Mann's Chinese Theater, the Hollywood Entertainment Museum, the Egyptian Theater, and the usual tourist franchises. There are many places to eat and at least one good wind-down restaurant/pub. |

The Hollywood Hills represent a rare opportunity in the heart of Los Angeles to escape from crowds and automobiles, while never being far from civilization. There are also many interesting attractions in the vicinity. After considerable research and first-hand exploring, we put together a route that meets all our criteria exceedingly well.

The route starts and ends on Hollywood Boulevard in the tourist precinct between Vine Street and Highland Avenue. Transport to and from here is a breeze—you simply take that modern Metro Red Line train from downtown or other Metro origins. This is also an interesting destination, with all the Hollywood tourist paraphernalia right there, plus eating and drinking establishments.

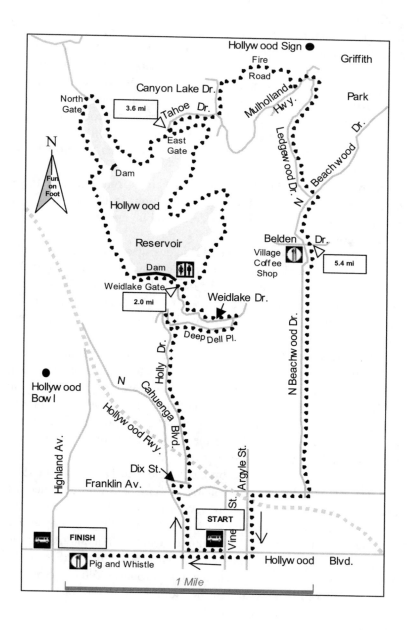

The route we suggest is 7.5 miles. There is probably too much uphill to call it a running route (for the average on-foot exerciser). It would be fairer to call it a part-running part-hiking/walking route. Most importantly, it covers very good on-foot terrain with no significant vehicle hazards and sufficient other on-foot people around to maintain a general sense of environmental comfort. Frankly, we were somewhat surprised at finding such a route that satisfied all our criteria so well in this city—the city with the most pedestrian-unfriendly reputation in the nation. Just one small caution: This route will not work on Thanksgiving, Christmas, or New Year's Day, when the Hollywood Reservoir is closed.

Start at Hollywood and Vine—you can alight from Red Line trains here, at one of the most classy subway stations in the country. The Hollywood and Vine Station is modern, well lit, and quite spectacular with its movie theme decoration.

Walk or run west on Hollywood Boulevard and turn right on North Cahuenga Boulevard. Go past Franklin Avenue one short block to Dix Street, turn right, and then go east one short block to Holly Drive. Now, take a deep breath. You have escaped from LA's automobile mania. From now on you will be on either vehicle-free paths or streets where cars are infrequent and travel slowly.

The next section (roughly one-and-a-half miles) is uphill. Proceed up Holly Drive to its end, follow a switchback to the right on Deep Dell Place, then take Weidlake Drive to the left, up to the Weidlake Gate of the Hollywood Reservoir. At this point you should be starting to feel good—there is a great view downward of the homes of Cahuenga Pass, and a great view upward of the deep blue and placid Hollywood Reservoir and its heavily treed environs.

The reservoir is supported by the Mulholland Dam, built in 1924 and dedicated to William Mulholland, the engineer who designed the Los Angeles drinking water supply system. There are restrooms here.

From this point, you have the luxury of proceeding on vehicle-free roads around the reservoir. The going is relatively flat and the footing sound, so this is good running terrain. We suggest proceeding to the reservoir's East Gate, using a choice of two routes. You can cross the dam and proceed clockwise past the North Gate to the East Gate, or just proceed anticlockwise to the East Gate. Either option is roughly 1.6 miles.

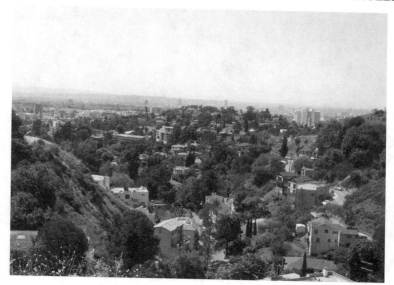

## Cahuenga Pass from the Hollywood Reservoir

Leave the reservoir at the East Gate and follow Tahoe Drive to Canyon Lake Drive, then turn left and continue uphill. You encounter an intersection where there is a trailhead on the right-hand side. By this point you have an excellent view of the Hollywood Sign just above you.

While many might consider this sign the ultimate in tacky-ness, at first hand it is, nevertheless, quite impressive. Constructed in 1923, the sign is 450 feet long and the letters are 50 feet tall. Thanks to Peggy Entwhistle, an aspiring actress who leapt to her death from the top of the "H" in 1932, you cannot now hike right to the sign. However, you get a great view of the sign from this trail.

Follow the trail—actually a fire road—to its end. This takes you across a virgin piece of Griffith Park to the residential Beachwood Canyon area, which you can traverse back down to Hollywood proper.

The trail exits somewhat curiously—you duck under a tree that seems to be in someone's front yard, and all of a sudden you are on Mulholland Highway. (This is the closest experience I have ever had to Paddington Station's Platform nine-and-a-half in Harry Potter.) You would not easily find the entrance to this trail if you were executing the route in the opposite direction.

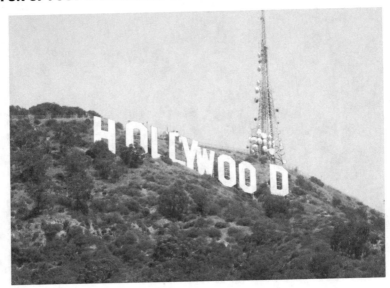

**The Hollywood Sign**

Mulholland Highway is itself a little curious—despite the grandiose name it is actually a quiet, winding, hilly suburban street.

Proceed uphill on Mulholland Highway, then take Ledgewood Drive to the right. From here on it is downhill all of the way back to Hollywood Boulevard—easy running or walking, as you feel inclined.

The area you have now entered is Hollywoodland, a famous real estate development from the 1920s. The Hollywood sign was erected as part of this development—the "land" letters were removed from the sign after the city took it over in the 1940s. Hollywoodland was home at various times to such celebrities as Doris Day, Vincent Price, Bugsy Siegel, Aldous Huxley, and Madonna. Humphrey Bogart used to live right here on Ledgewood Drive, an attractive winding street lined by quite classy hillside houses.[2]

Ledgewood takes you to N Beachwood Drive, which you follow thereafter. At Belden Drive you find the Village Coffee Shop, an excellent stop for breakfast or lunch (but no alcohol). This is at the commercial center of the Hollywoodland development.

---

2        Source: http://www.laconservancy.org/initiatives/
HOLLYWOODLAND.pdf

Continue down Beachwood to Franklin Avenue. Use the ordinary streets to get back to Hollywood and Vine (for example, via Franklin, Argyle, and Hollywood).

Hollywood Boulevard is not what it was in the 1920s or 1930s. Today there are many touristy things to see, mainly a little westward, around Hollywood and Highland. Walking there from Hollywood and Vine you will pass various attractions and eating-places.

When Nola and I were there, after our run-hike we settled on the Pig and Whistle restaurant and bar for our wind-down. The food was good and the bar friendly. The Pig and Whistle is next to Grauman's Egyptian Theatre at Las Palmas Avenue. The restaurant is styled similarly to the theatre. They were both restored in 2001 to reflect the Art Deco style of the 1927 original. In Hollywood's *Golden Age*, Spencer Tracy, Loretta Young, Howard Hughes, Barbara Stanwyck, and many other stars visited this restaurant.

Continue along Hollywood to Highland. Here you find the Hollywood & Highland mega-entertainment complex, which includes the Kodak Theater, home of the Academy Awards presentations. After you have seen enough, you can catch the Red Line Train here back to downtown Los Angeles or other transit transfer points.

# UCLA to Santa Monica

| | |
|---|---|
| **Distance** | 7.3 miles |
| **Comfort** | Good running or walking conditions. Roughly half the route is along the edges or center strip of a particularly wide street with grassy side trails (San Vicente Boulevard). The other half is along regular street sidewalks. The route is generally flat. Expect plenty of people and automobile traffic around. Not recommended for inline skating. |
| **Attractions** | The main attractions are the two end-points, a major California college campus and a beautiful and lively ocean-side resort city. The route in between, while not spectacular, is generally very pleasant. |
| **Convenience** | Start at UCLA and end in Santa Monica. Both points are linked to each other via Big Blue Bus Lines 1, 2, 3, or 8, and to downtown Los Angeles via the Metro Rapid 720 express bus. This route also works well in the opposite direction. |
| **Destination** | Santa Monica, with its beach, pier, amusement park, and abundant restaurant, bar, and shopping selections. If starting from Santa Monica, the destination is the attractive UCLA campus. Either way, there is convenient public transit back to the start point via Big Blue or Metro bus. |

This route works either way. If you are staying or living near the UCLA campus, this route represents an excellent way to get to the beautiful beaches and surrounding attractions of Santa Monica. Alternatively, if you happen to be staying in one of Santa Monica's hotels and feel the need to see what lies inland, this is a great way to explore UCLA and other places in that direction.

This route exploits San Vicente Boulevard, a street that represents a major anomaly in the design of the Los Angeles regional road system. San Vicente, for most of its length, is a wide, pleasant, tree-lined road, including a center nature strip with paths for pedestrians. Vehicle traffic is moderate and there are generally plenty of other on-foot exercisers around.

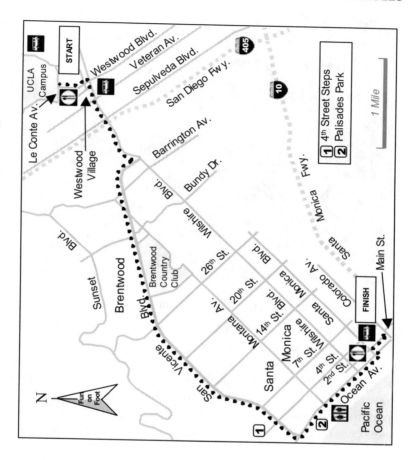

We describe the route in the direction UCLA to Santa Monica. We nominally start at the intersection of Le Conte Avenue and Westwood Boulevard, where the UCLA campus meets lively Westwood Village.

Follow Westwood Avenue past the village shops and other establishments to Wilshire Boulevard. Turn right on Wilshire. This takes you past the Los Angeles National Cemetery, under the San Diego Freeway, and into the Veterans Administration area. Take the first major road to the right, which becomes San Vicente Avenue.

The first part of San Vicente is very commercial in nature. However, the character becomes more residential as you progress westward. You pass the Brentwood Country Club on the left.

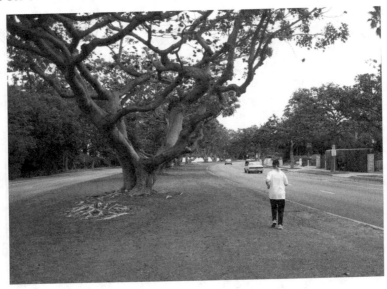

### San Vicente Avenue, Santa Monica

At 26th Street, you cross the Los Angeles-Santa Monica boundary. From this point on, the environment is entirely residential. The on-foot conditions are excellent, with a choice of using either sidewalk or the grassy center strip. You encounter more on-foot exercisers now. However, there are no restrooms after 26th Street until you reach the oceanfront—a typical consequence of on-footing in residential areas anywhere. If needed, you can find a restroom at the gas station at 26th Street.

Follow San Vicente to 4th Street. If you divert to the right here, you come to the 4th Street Steps, 189 steps up a steep incline and a popular place for local fitness buffs to gain exercise and public exposure.

Continue along San Vicente to Ocean Avenue. Turn left onto Ocean Avenue, following the beach reserve called Palisades Park into central Santa Monica. There are public restrooms in the park.

As described in our first route, there are many eating and drinking places for winding down in central Santa Monica. If you turn left into Santa Monica Boulevard, you find Ye Olde King's Head Restaurant and Pub just before 2nd Street. Continue a further short block and you are in the middle of Third Street Promenade, a pedestrian precinct with numerous shops and additional eating-places.

To take a bus back to UCLA you have a choice of Big Blue Bus lines: Line 1 or 8 (catch in Santa Monica Boulevard or Main Street) or Line 2 or 3 (catch in 4th Street).

This route works equally well in the reverse direction. At the UCLA end, there are various eating-places in Westwood Village, between the Westwood and Wilshire intersection and the UCLA campus at Le Conte Avenue. A good place to wind down is Jerry's Famous Deli in Weyburn Avenue, off Westwood Boulevard a short block south of Le Conte. Jerry's has an enormous menu including breakfasts, salads, sandwiches, and a wide choice of entrees, all of the above at all hours. Prices are modest and the place is very popular. Beer and wine are available. There are also various other places to eat nearby, including fast food and some mid- and up-scale restaurants.

You can also explore the UCLA campus. A run or walk around the campus perimeter is a fine idea if you feel like doing a further four miles with a few moderate grades.

To take a bus back to Santa Monica, catch a Big Blue Bus (any of Lines 1, 2, 3, or 8) at Westwood and Le Conte.

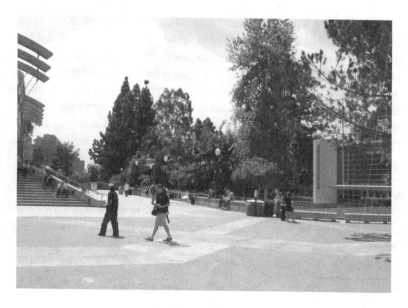

**UCLA Campus**

# Other Ideas

In our first route we covered what we consider LA's best five-to-six-mile beachside route, generally following the **South Bay Bicycle Trail**. That trail also extends a further 13.6 miles southward from Marina Del Rey's Fisherman's Village.[3] It passes through Dockweiler Beach—if you like aircraft, you'll experience plenty of them around here, landing or taking off at LAX airport. It then passes through El Porto Beach, Manhattan Beach, Hermosa Beach, King Harbor, and Redondo Beach, ending at Torrance Beach. Depending on just where you are staying, this presents you with a large number of interesting on-foot route possibilities. The trail also extends northward from Santa Monica Pier roughly three miles to Will Rogers Beach.

Another area where we have run is the unique residential suburb of **Beverly Hills**. It is a pleasant residential environment for the on-foot exerciser and, if you are so inclined, you can craft routes that take you past homes of famous people. (Stars' homes maps are available at most tourist outlets.) There is even a guided running tour that passes various celebrities' homes.[4]

We tried hard to find a nice on-foot route close to downtown Los Angeles, where so many visitors stay. The obvious choice is **Elysian Park**, roughly two miles north of downtown. We were excited by a reference in a popular runners' magazine to the idea of running around Dodgers Stadium and parts of Elysian Park, starting and ending downtown. After spending a very long day trying to make this work, we ended disappointed. First, the surroundings on the way to the Dodgers Stadium vicinity were decidedly seedy. Then, when entering Elysian Park, the environment improved but on-foot travel was limited to road edges—no sidewalks. Inside Elysian Park, there were indications of interesting trails, but attempts to find the best ones proved challenging. Maps are elusive (the only official we could find told us we would have to go to the rangers' station at Griffith Park, a few miles away and accessible only by automobile). Furthermore, there were not enough other on-footers around to keep the comfort factor high enough. When returning to downtown via the northeasterly perimeter of Dodgers

---

3        For a full map of the trail refer to: http://www.scc.ca.gov/Wheel/lapage/2_smb/bike.html
4        Not having tried this, we cannot explicitly recommend it. However, more information is available at: http://www.offnrunningtours.com/

Stadium, we again found ourselves in a quite seedy environment (barred windows on all houses do not inspire confidence). If you want to venture into this area on-foot, we strongly encourage you do so only in the company of a local who knows exactly where to go.

Another area we researched was **Griffith Park**, a large green space about six miles northwest of downtown and adjacent to the Hollywood Hills area described in our second route. However, we did not succeed in satisfying our convenience and destination criteria. If you don't mind driving to Griffith Park, there are several options for an on-foot outing. Detailed information on running/hiking/walking trails in the park is not easy to find in advance. We found the Park Rangers very helpful though, so you might want to drop by their office on Crystal Springs Drive for information and a map.

The Los Angeles region is so enormous that we have no doubt there are many other excellent on-foot routes around. We look forward to hearing from readers about routes that meet all of our selection criteria.

* * * *

Los Angeles is a fascinating city, with plenty to see, an ideal climate for outdoors activities, excellent beaches, and, of course, the ever-present entertainment industry culture. Parts of the region, at least, fit our fun-on-foot model well. There is no shortage of attractions and destinations. Comfort can be good, subject to judicious selection of routes from the safety angle. Convenience demands can be satisfied, thanks to a generally good public transit system.

LA's attachment to the automobile is somewhat at odds with the fun-on-foot mentality. However, provided you understand the driving style, you can usually work around that little problem.

Having lived so long in Boston, I found the difference between Boston and LA drivers particularly striking. To sum up the difference: *Boston drivers stop for pedestrians but not red lights. LA drivers stop for red lights but not pedestrians.*

Enjoy Southern California and have fun on foot in and around Los Angeles!

# 15

# America's Finest City

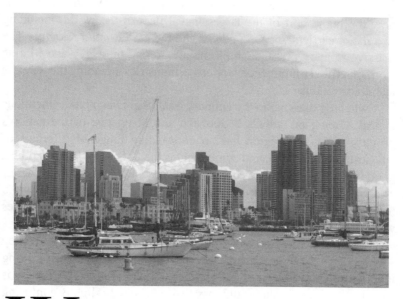

While I don't necessarily buy the "finest city" bit—a daring creation of the city's marketing folk—San Diego is indeed a great place. Famous for its zoo, beaches, Navy and Marine Corps bases, sea craft, and golf, it also has much to offer the on-foot exerciser.

The number one quality is the weather, which many claim is the best in the United States. The statistics support this claim. San Diego's average maximum *and* minimum temperatures lie within our preferred range of 40-to-80 degrees Fahrenheit in *every month* of the year. Furthermore, on average, there is precipitation on only 42 days per year

(12%), and 147 days (41%) are brilliantly cloudless. You don't get a better climate for outdoor on-foot exercise anywhere!

San Diego also has its share of history to build into on-foot route planning. This city, located on the site of California's first European settlement, is considered the birthplace of California. In 1542, Juan Rodríguez Cabrillo sailed into San Diego Bay and claimed the land for Spain. Spanish civilization started here in 1769. In 1822, the city came under Mexican jurisdiction, when Mexico gained its independence. In the U.S.-Mexican War in 1846, the city was captured by the United States.

San Diego became an important naval base in World War I. It is now the home port of the largest naval fleet in the world, including two major carriers, the *USS Nimitz* and the *USS Ronald Reagan*. The massive military presence, built mainly around the Navy and Marine Corps, has bred a number of supportive industries including the wireless technology industry.

Switching thinking to the culinary train, San Diego has tremendous appeal. Being on Mexico's doorstep and being one of the nation's primary ports, this region has an outstanding range of offerings of Mexican food, seafood, and combinations thereof. The idea of ending a good day out on-foot at an eating establishment works very well here.

Considering the safety factor, the violent crime rate index is 5.8 (crimes per 1,000 residents in 2003). This is the best figure for all cities we cover.

Public transit in San Diego is a mixed bag. There is the Trolley service (a light rail system) to selected areas, a bus network serving inner areas generally, and train services to outer areas. The Trolley is excellent—clean, frequent, and easy to use. The only slightly confusing thing is that all the services, which include the Blue Line, Orange Line, and Green Line, use vehicles that are painted bright red! We can forgive that eccentricity. If one has a complaint about the trolley system, it is the limitation in the territory it covers.

The bus service is a different story. We would have to grade it one of the worst in the U.S. cities we have visited. It seems designed purely to meet the needs of local commuters, without consideration for city visitors or those locals who don't have or want to use a car to get around in leisure hours. The schedules outside commuter peak hours and on weekends are abysmal, and service is unreliable. We waited over an hour for a 30-minute-frequency bus at one point, then the bus was crowded and the driver unapologetic and unfriendly. There were no paper system maps anywhere in the city, and we were told there would be none for three months. Maybe we were just unlucky, but I suspect the problems in this transit system go deep.

The longer-range train service is not very frequent outside commuter hours, but that is more forgivable since it is overtly a commuter service. We did find the trains spotless and pleasant to ride.

The bottom line transit-wise is that this city operates on the common Californian assumption that everyone drives a vehicle to get anywhere, unless highway congestion or parking costs force otherwise.

\* \* \* \*

Taking the above background into account, and scanning the map of the region around downtown, a few areas stand out as prospectively great on-foot exercise areas:   the ocean shore (almost anywhere), Mission Bay, the San Diego River, and Balboa Park (a major recreation reserve close to downtown).   Nola and I spent a lot of time exploring (usually with big smiles on our faces) these and some other prospective routes.   We ended up pinning down four routes that we believe capture the best overall qualities for an on-foot exerciser who is staying in or near downtown San Diego.

| Route | Distance |
|---|---|
| 1.  Balboa Park | 5.5 miles |
| 2.  San Diego Bay | 3.9 miles |
| 3.  Sea World and Old Town | 6.5 miles |
| 4.  Mission Bay, Mission Beach, and Old Town | 10.6 miles |

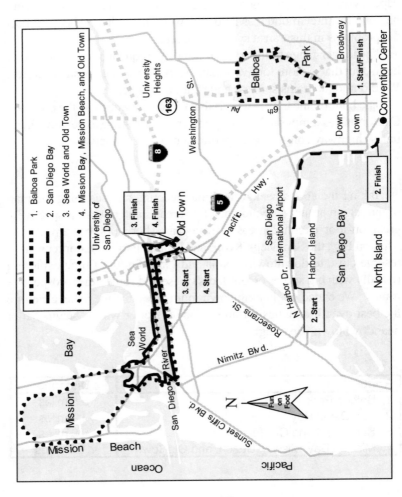

**San Diego Routes**

# Balboa Park

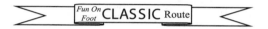

| Distance | 5.5 miles |
|---|---|
| Comfort | Mainly dedicated pedestrian or pedestrian/bicycle trails inside the park, and good street sidewalks otherwise. You have a choice of level, paved trails or more adventurous terrain. Expect plenty of other on-footers around any day. Crowds are unlikely to be a concern. Not suitable for inline skating. |
| Attractions | A beautiful nature preserve, providing escape from city life. Experience a variety of native plant environments, ranging from canyons to wildflower fields. You also pass by Balboa Park's other attractions such as the San Diego Zoo, several major museums, and various cultural venues. |
| Convenience | Start and end at 6th Avenue and C Street in downtown San Diego, on the Trolley line and less than a mile on-foot from the Convention Center and major hotels. |
| Destination | Finish downtown on the threshold of the Gaslamp Quarter, San Diego's premier eating, drinking, and entertainment area. Alternatively, consider the Balboa Park museum precinct your destination, take in the places that are for you, and have a short walk back downtown afterwards. |

For folks staying downtown and in need of an hour-or-two break, this is an easy and very pleasant escape from city life. No cars or public transit are needed. It is also convenient to Trolley routes.

Balboa Park is San Diego's answer to Central Park—big, green, pleasant, popular, and close to downtown. It has been instrumental in getting San Diego on the international map. It was the site of the 1915-16 Panama-California Exposition, commemorating the opening of the Panama Canal. It was also the site of the 1935-36 California Pacific International Exposition, held to boost the local economy during the Great Depression. These events are attributed with creating most of

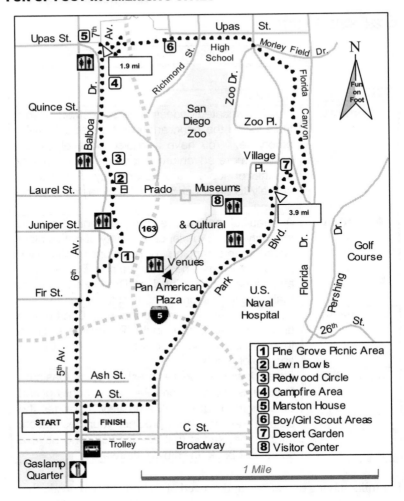

the magnificent Spanish Colonial Revival buildings that now house museums in the park.

Balboa Park is an excellent place for on-foot exercise. You can easily run or walk to the park from downtown hotels or the Trolley. You then have a choice of underfoot terrain, ranging from flat paved pedestrian/ bicycle trails, to sunny, hilly paths through fields of wildflowers, to steep wilderness trails in canyons. When you have had enough of that, there are various places to end up, including the impressive collection of museums right in the park. For an eating or drinking wind-down session, you are but a skip and a jump from San Diego's prime eating and drinking area—the Gaslamp Quarter.

We nominally start and end at C Street and 6th Avenue, on the Trolley Blue and Orange Lines and no more than a mile on foot from the Convention Center and the main hotels.

Go north on 6th Street to Fir Street. Take the path to the right here, up and into the park. Cross the first road and keep going towards the Pine Grove picnic tables. Pick up the paved trail heading north.

---

**VARIATION**

Instead of taking the paved trail north, you can use a lower trail through the ravine along the Route 163 highway. This is a much wilder trail, further away from people and closer to the rest of nature. However, underfoot conditions are not so good, the trail is much steeper, and there is always the intruding noise of the highway traffic. You will find paths down to this trail at various points.

---

Keep following the trail northward. Pass the Juniper Street park entrance, where there are restrooms. Continue up to El Prado, a major entrance road to the park's museum area, via the Cabrillo Bridge across the ravine. (You will have an opportunity to visit the museum area later.) Cross El Prado, and continue following the trail northward past the lawn bowling and Redwood Circle. Cross Quince Drive and continue past the campfire area. In due course, you will see the Marston House high-rise ahead.

As you approach Marston House, bear right and take the trail heading down into the canyon. You need to descend to a pedestrian bridge across the creek and the Route 163 highway. The trail here is not paved and it gets a little steep in parts. However, these conditions do not last for long.

After crossing the bridge, follow the trail upwards. The trail exits onto the sidewalk of Upas Street, the northern boundary of Balboa Park. Pass the Boy Scouts and Girl Scouts areas and the Roosevelt Jr. High School. Continue to the intersection with Park Boulevard.

Go south one short block to Morley Field Drive. You here have a choice of routes. If you want to experience some different terrain and are not committed to the fastest route, we recommend a trek over the hillsides along Florida Canyon (also known as Powerhouse Canyon).

Cross to the southeastern corner of the intersection and keep going southeast. You come to a little trailhead. The trail heads south away from the road.

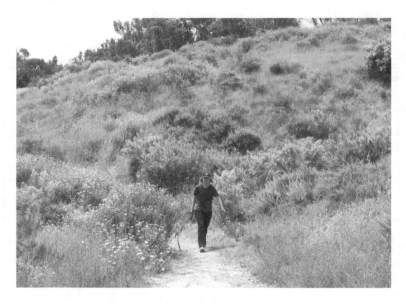

**Nola in Sunny Florida Canyon**

**VARIATION**

There is a paved, level alternative to the hillside trek, which is faster and easier. Simply follow the western sidewalk of Park Boulevard southward to the museum precinct, and then pick up our main route again there.

Follow the trail south through the field. We have found it very beautiful here in the spring, with all the wildflowers in bloom. There are some grades and potholes but nothing extreme. You might wish to consider this part as a hike, although we encountered several fit folk running through here.

As you approach the road called Zoo Place and see the intersection with busy Florida Drive below, we suggest you keep bearing right and take the uphill path to intersect Zoo Place. Cross Zoo Place and pick up the paved zigzag trail up the hill here.

---

**VARIATION**

You can trek down to the Florida Drive intersection, cross Florida Drive, and pick up the southbound trail following Florida Drive on its east side to Pershing Drive. From here you can exit the park via 26th Street. Then, from 26th Street, turn right into B Street or C Street to get back to central downtown. This variation lengthens the route by roughly a mile and avoids the more populous part of the park around the museums and other institutions. However, the going is rougher and there can be heavy vehicle traffic on Florida Drive.

---

Continue up the zigzag trail and emerge in the Desert Garden. What a pleasant surprise! The Desert Garden is spectacular with its display of cacti of numerous colors, shapes and sizes. Proceed through the Desert Garden and take the footbridge over Park Boulevard to the museum area.

Museums here include the Museum of Man, Museum of Art, Natural History Museum, Automotive Museum, Aerospace Museum, and Sports Museum. Take this opportunity to visit any of them if you wish. There are not many quality casual restaurants here, but there are places to grab a snack and a soda.

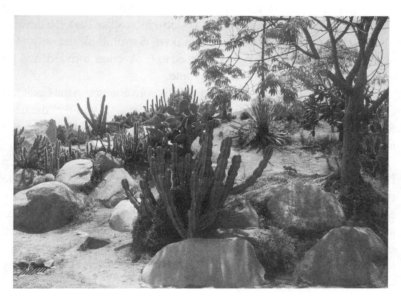

**The Desert Garden in Balboa Park**

---

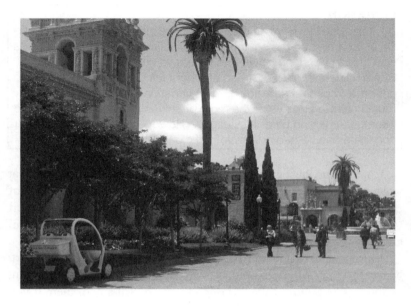

**Balboa Park Museum Precinct**

To get from the museum precinct to central downtown or the Convention Center, simply take the western sidewalk of Park Boulevard. This leads you quickly back to downtown, downhill all the way. Go down to A Street and turn right. Proceed to 6th Avenue, turn left, and go on to C Street where we started the route.

One reason we chose this end point is its convenience to the Gaslamp Quarter, San Diego's top eating and drinking area. If you feel the need for a wind-down meal or drink, go one block west and then turn left into 5th Avenue.

There are many fine establishments in the strip of 5th Avenue between Broadway and K Street. We sampled several places here. Our favorite is The Field Irish Restaurant and Pub at 544 5th Avenue, just south of Market Street. The Field, with an interior shipped from Ireland, is as authentically Irish as any pub outside Ireland. Our server explained how even the staff mostly came from Ireland. This establishment has an excellent Irish and traditional food menu, with evening and Sunday afternoon entertainment to boot.

# San Diego Bay

| Distance | 3.9 miles |
|---|---|
| Comfort | A dedicated, paved pedestrian or pedestrian/ bicycle trail all the way, with plenty of other pedestrians around. The last mile might become crowded at busy tourist times. OK for inline skating. |
| Attractions | San Diego's maritime highlights, including views of sea craft on the bay and moored at Harbor Island. Also see historic Spanish Landing, the historic ships of the Maritime Museum (including the *Star of India*, the world's oldest active ship), and the *USS Midway*, which houses the Aircraft Carrier Museum. |
| Convenience | Start at Spanish Landing, about four miles northeast of central downtown. There is a direct bus (Route 922 or 923) here from downtown on weekdays and a Trolley-plus-bus (Route 28) connection via Old Town every day. End downtown near the Convention Center. |
| Destination | Finish at Seaport Village, just north of the Convention Center. There are shops, entertainment, and some nice wind-down restaurant/bars at Seaport Village, or pick your own favorite downtown destination. |

One of San Diego's most exciting characteristics is its bond to the maritime world, both military and civilian. Not only is the city host to the largest naval fleet in the world, but it is also a major commercial port, fishing port, and hub of recreational sailing. We felt we must include an on-foot route along San Diego Bay, the maritime heart of San Diego.

If you are staying downtown and simply want a short run up and back on the bay shore, that is straightforward and does not need my directions. We have another suggestion, however, which avoids the out-and-back characteristic that all too often results in us cutting our route short. ("I think I've had enough now—I'll turn back.")

We suggest taking a bus out along the bay shore then running, jogging, or walking back to downtown. This route has most of the characteristics we always seek. There is only one caveat—a less-than-ideal bus service to the start-point. On weekdays, there is a direct bus from downtown, albeit with a 45-minute frequency. On weekends, your best option is a Trolley-to-bus transfer through Old Town. Bus routes and schedules change from time-to-time, of course, so you should check these details out at the time.

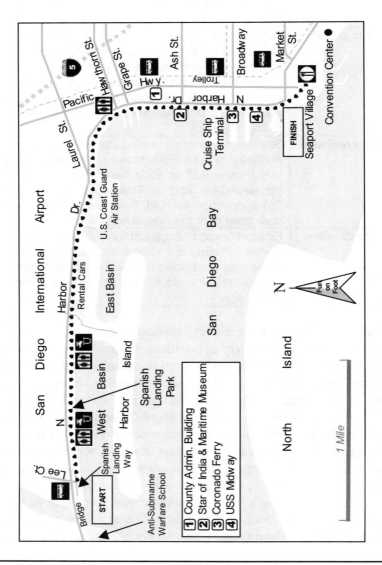

Our route starts at Spanish Landing, a historic location and a very pleasant park. To get to Spanish Landing via public transit, we know of two options. First, on weekdays only, catch a Route 922 or 923 bus in Broadway (westbound) or North Harbor Drive (northbound). Check a timetable (available online) before starting out for the bus stop.[1] Take the bus past the airport. Alight on North Harbor Drive at the intersection signposted "Spanish Landing Way/Lee Ct." Cross the main road and enter Spanish Landing Park.

The other option, which works all days but takes longer, is to catch the Trolley Blue Line to Old Town, and connect to a Route 28 bus. Alight on Rosecrans Street at the intersection with Nimitz Boulevard. Head southeast on Nimitz to its intersection with North Harbor Drive. Cross the latter to the front gate of the Fleet Anti-Submarine Warfare Training Center. Then head east, cross the bridge, and enter Spanish Landing Park.

---

**VARIATION**

You can tack on a little extra to the front of this route by starting at Point Loma around Shelter Island Drive and passing through the Sport Fishing Pier area. The underfoot conditions are not so good on that part of the route, but you get to see more sea craft and a lively part of the city. Take the Route 28 bus from Old Town. Stay on the bus on Rosecrans Street past Nimitz Boulevard and alight a few blocks later at Dickens Street or Byron Street. Go a block southeast to Scott Street. Head east bearing right, close to the waterfront. This takes you to the sidewalk of North Harbor Drive. Follow that sidewalk past the Anti-Submarine Warfare Training Center and over the bridge to Spanish Landing Park.

---

Spanish Landing is where the *San Antonio* dropped anchor in 1769. It was the first ship to arrive as part of a multi-pronged expedition led by Captain Gaspar de Portola, Governor of California. The goal of the expedition was to settle the San Diego area and points north in California. It led to the establishment, a couple of months later, of the first mission on Presidio Hill near Old Town San Diego.

Follow the paved pedestrian trail through Spanish Landing Park. In parts, bicycles have their own path, but sometimes they share the

---

1     The San Diego transit website is at: http://www.sdcommute.com/

pedestrian trail.  Enjoy views of the mass of sea craft moored at Harbor Island across the basin.

As you approach Harbor Island Drive, the access road to Harbor Island from North Harbor Drive, the trail splits.  You have the choice of bearing left along North Harbor Drive or bearing right onto Harbor Island.  The latter, while very pleasant, is actually a dead end.  We therefore suggest taking the left-hand path.  Cross Harbor Island Drive at the light.

For the next mile, the route is less pleasant.  There is still a good paved trail underfoot, but you are flanked on the left by busy North Harbor Drive and the airport beyond it and on the right by facilities that keep you away from the waterfront.  First there is the collection of airport rental car facilities that rudely impose themselves on an otherwise very nice area.  After that, there is the U.S. Coast Guard Air Station, which also separates you from the water.

After the Coast Guard station, everything improves immensely. The trail follows the shore and the scenery becomes very attractive. The density of people on the trail also increases, as you get closer to downtown.  This part of the bay is known as Embarcadero Crescent.

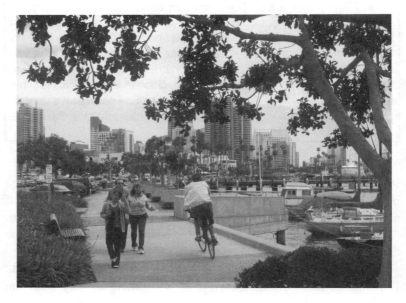

**Embarcadero Crescent Trail Approaching Downtown**

Pass the distinctive County Administration Building. You then come to the Maritime Museum, and its collection of tall ships right on the trail. The most prominent vessel is the *Star of India*, launched in 1863, and the world's oldest active ship. There are several other historic vessels moored here, including a Soviet attack submarine. You can tour these ships.

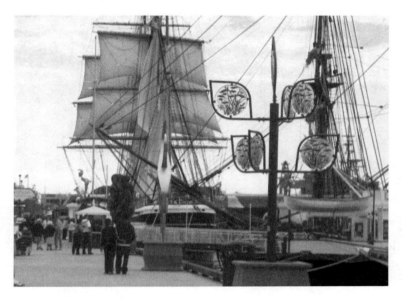

**Maritime Museum Ships Including the *Star of India***

Continuing southward, you pass several docks. After the cruise ship terminal is Navy Pier. Moored here is the now-decommissioned *USS Midway*. Commissioned in 1945 and in active duty for 47 years, this carrier served in battles from WWII through to Desert Storm in 1991. It now acts as host of the San Diego Aircraft Carrier Museum—well worth seeing if you have the time.

If you continue south from here you come to Seaport Village, where we end our nominal route. Seaport Village is a tourist destination, with shops, entertainment, fast food outlets, and a couple of restaurant/bars. It is a fine place to wind-down from an on-foot outing. We settled down to a good lunch at the Edgewater Grill, a lovely waterfront restaurant with a dining patio right on the water.

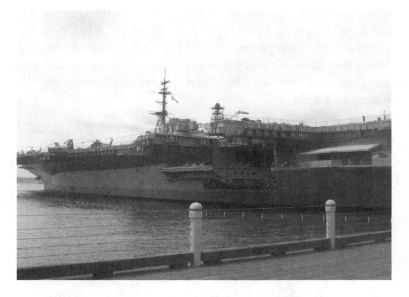

*USS Midway*—Now the San Diego Aircraft Carrier Museum

Here you are very convenient to the Convention Center, downtown hotels, the Trolley line, and the Gaslamp Quarter.

# Sea World and Old Town

| Distance | 6.5 miles |
|---|---|
| Comfort | Most of the route is along dedicated pedestrian/ bicycle trails. In some parts, you need to follow street sidewalks, and there are a few busy streets to cross. If it is a nice day, expect other pedestrians or cyclists around. OK for inline skating. |
| Attractions | The San Diego River banks with their extensive bird life, the Quivira Basin marinas, and Sea World. End in historic Old Town San Diego. |
| Convenience | Start and end in Old Town, three-to-four miles north of central downtown. This point can be conveniently reached via the comfortable and frequent San Diego Trolley Blue Line. |
| Destination | Old Town San Diego State Historic Park is a restored and reconstructed collection of buildings and their surrounds that recapture the nineteenth century spirit of the city's oldest precinct. There are museums, shops, restaurants, and bars. There is much to see, good food, and convenient transport back downtown. |

This route will be especially appealing to the visitor to San Diego who wants to see the sights and get some on-foot exercise at the same time. In particular, if you want to visit Shamu at Sea World and also explore Old Town San Diego, this route is a winner!

This route starts and ends in Old Town, one of the most interesting parts of San Diego historically and also an excellent place for a food and beverage wind-down. Furthermore, one can easily get between Old Town and downtown hotels via the Trolley.

Start from the Old Town Transit Center, where the Trolley Blue Line and the Coaster Trains that serve northern regions stop. Head northwest and cross Taylor Street. Turn right onto the sidewalk of Pacific Highway. If you like the idea of a breakfast before starting out, you will pass a very popular breakfast place, Perry's Café, on this road.

Continue following Pacific Highway a short distance to just before the river bridge. Here you find a trailhead giving access to the paved bicycle path that follows the southern bank of the San Diego River. Turn left, heading westward or downstream.

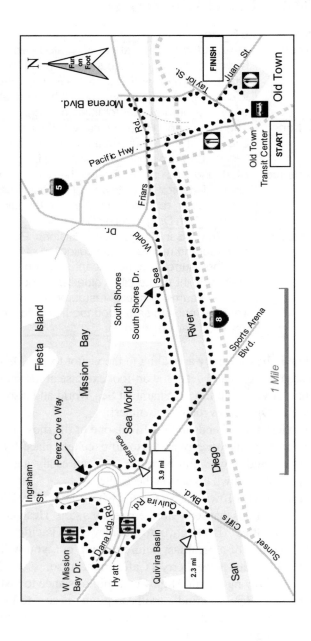

The San Diego River is not stunningly beautiful, to say the least. The river itself is usually quite narrow and what you see is more an accompanying floodway. However, there is a lot of interesting bird life here, the trail is excellent, and this is a great way to connect on-foot to the Mission Bay and Sea World area.

Follow the trail to the Sports Arena Boulevard Bridge. Go up to street level and take the bridge sidewalk across the river. Go down to the riverside trail on the northern bank and head west. Pass the next bridge (the Sunset Cliffs Boulevard Bridge) and then leave the trail heading northward. Cross Quivira Road and enter the marina area.

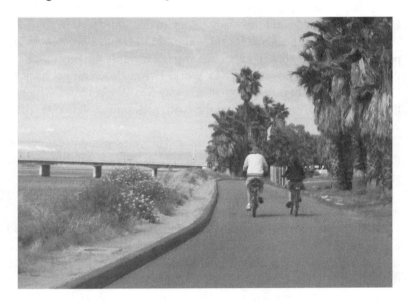

**The Riverside Trail**

The Quivira Basin and its marinas constitute a very pleasant part of the route. On-footers can run, jog, or walk around the marina edge, ogle the amazing sea craft docked here, and be entertained by the sea lions on the barges. There are various facilities for food and drink, and public restrooms at the back of the Seaforth Marina. Bicycles and inline skates are not allowed—if you are an inline skater, follow the sidewalk of Quivira Road instead.

Just before the Hyatt resort, there is a street off to the right. This takes you to W Mission Bay Drive. Cross W Mission Bay Drive and you come to Dana Landing Road. To negotiate the Dana Landing area you have a choice of paths. You can bear left and pick up the trail following Mission Bay towards the north and east. Alternatively, follow the path along Dana Landing Road. Either way, you end up at the intersection of Dana Landing Road and Ingraham Street.

Cross Ingraham Street at the light and continue straight ahead into Perez Cove Way. Pick up the bike trail on the west side of Perez Cove Way. Follow the paved bike trail around Sea World. If you have the time and the inclination, drop in to see Shamu and the other sights Sea World offers.

At one point the marked trail crosses back to the left side of Perez Cove Way at a pedestrian crossing. Stick to that trail for now.

When you get past Sea World and close to South Shores, you are presented with a choice of either bearing left towards the Bay or taking the pedestrian crossing across Sea World Drive. You can get back to Old Town either way. We suggest crossing Sea World Drive, which is the shorter route. After crossing the road, pick up the shared driving/walking/bicycle road along the river.

I know that sharing a road with cars and bicycles sounds a dangerous thing for pedestrians. However, it works here. This is an old two-lane street, which now leads nowhere. Therefore, vehicles are quite rare here, and any vehicle would not be in a hurry to go anywhere. Therefore, it turns out to be a winning deal for pedestrians and cyclists.

Take the shared road eastward to its end. There, pedestrians can find a little path onto the southern sidewalk of Friars Road.

Follow the Friars Road sidewalk under overpasses for Interstate 5, the Pacific Highway, then two rail bridges (for trains and the Trolley respectively). You need to cross Friars Road somewhere here. There is not a lot of traffic but vehicles do move fast, so be careful. In some spots there is a wide center strip for staging in the middle of the road and good visibility in both directions.

Having got to the north side of Friars Road past the rail track overpasses, climb the first set of concrete steps up from the road. They take you to the western sidewalk of the next bridge—Morena Boulevard. Cross this bridge over Friars Road and the river. Continue along the sidewalk to Taylor Street, cross that street, and turn right. Turn left on Juan Street. Your destination—Old Town San Diego State Historic Park—appears on your right.

Old Town is where Father Junipero Serra came more than 225 years ago to establish the very first mission in a chain of 21 missions that were to be the cornerstones of California's Spanish colonization.

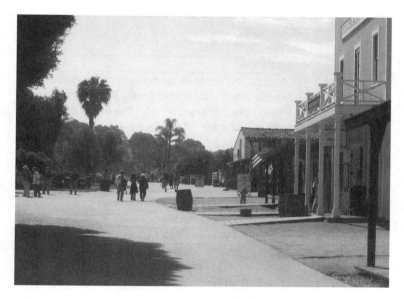

## Old Town State Historic Park

There are many interesting places to see here, including restored or replica houses, businesses, and schoolhouse. There are several museums. Admission is free. After entering the park in either Wallace Street or Garden Street, you come to a visitor center where you can pick up a helpful map and further information.

There are many good wind-down eating and drinking establishments in Old Town. Mexican restaurants stand out here, but there are other cuisine choices too. You can also continue through the historic park southeastward to San Diego Avenue, where there are more restaurant choices. Nola and I have tried several places and our favorite is Rancho Nopal Restaurant and Cantina, which happens to be one of the first places you will find, in Wallace Street next to the visitor center. This restaurant is decorated in classical Mexican style and has a pleasant outdoor patio. The menu offers a variety of Mexican food choices.

To get back to downtown, the Trolley is handy at the Transit Center on Congress Street near Taylor Street.

# Mission Bay, Mission Beach, and Old Town

NOTE: You need to refer to our Sea World and Old Town route description for directions for parts of this route.

| Distance | 10.6 miles |
| --- | --- |
| Comfort | Most of the route is along dedicated pedestrian/ bicycle trails. In some parts, it is necessary to follow street sidewalks, and there are a few busy streets to cross. If it is a nice day, expect other pedestrians or cyclists around. The Mission Beach area might be very crowded on a busy day, but you have the option of avoiding the beach and following the bay shore instead. OK for inline skating. |
| Attractions | Pass through a variety of very attractive areas, including the San Diego River banks, the Quivira Basin marinas, Mission Beach, and the western half of Mission Bay. Pass Sea World on the return loop and end in historic Old Town San Diego. |
| Convenience | Start and end in Old Town, three-to-four miles north of central downtown. This point can be conveniently reached via the comfortable and frequent San Diego Trolley Blue Line. |
| Destination | Old Town San Diego State Historic Park is a restored and reconstructed collection of buildings and their surrounds that recapture the nineteenth century spirit of the city's oldest precinct. There are museums, shops, restaurants, and bars. There is much to see, good food, and convenient transport back downtown. |

This route pulls together several very appealing parts of San Diego. If you were a stranger to town and had but one spare afternoon to get out and experience the city's outdoors offerings, this is what you absolutely should do.

This route follows most of the previous route, but additionally links in trails along popular Mission Beach and around the western half of scenic Mission Bay. This route starts and ends in Old Town.

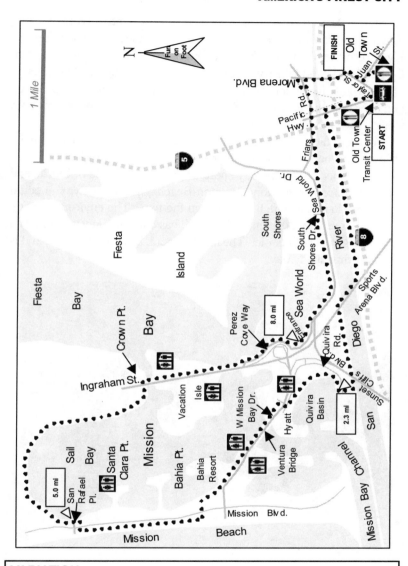

## VARIATION

If you have a car you can choose to omit Old Town and the river, and just do a loop of Mission Bay West and Mission Beach. Start and finish at the Quivira Basin marinas, where there is parking. Total loop distance is roughly four miles.

Start at the Old Town Transit Center. Follow our Sea World and Old Town route, past the Quivira Basin marinas, to the street just before the Hyatt resort leading to W Mission Bay Drive. Here we diverge from the Sea World and Old Town route, to take in the loop of Mission Bay.

Turn left, following either sidewalk of W Mission Bay Drive up and over the Ventura Bridge. After the bridge, there are restrooms both sides. Pass the Bahia Resort hotel.

You now face a fundamental choice as to the route to follow up the strip of land between the ocean and the western edge of Mission Bay. You can either follow the bay shore or go west a couple of blocks and follow the oceanfront along Mission Beach. Alternatively, you could choose to do some switching between the two. The environments on both sides are very different. The beach has crashing waves, wind, and sometimes loads of people. The bay is placid, has fewer people, and is pleasant almost any day.

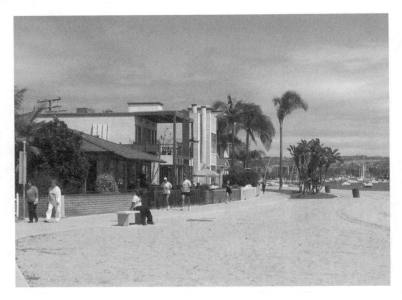

### The Bayside Trail, Mission Bay West

Let us assume you choose a mix. After the Bahia, bear right to the pedestrian path around the cove, and follow that as far as you want. When ready, pick a street to the left and cut through to the beach. There is a paved path the length of the beach, and plenty to see in the way of sand, surfers, bikinis, and happy people. Proceed north to San Raphael Place or an earlier cross street or alley. Cut back eastward to the bay trail.

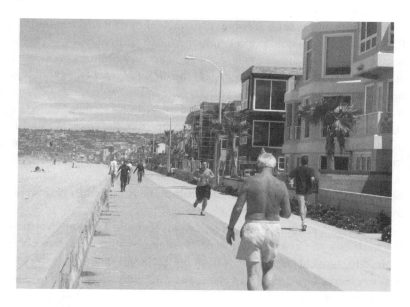

**Mission Beach Pedestrian Path on a Quiet Day**

Now follow the scenic Mission Bay trail around towards the east, then the south. You pass a major small craft sailing area on the way. Continue to Ingraham Street at the southern tip of Crown Point. Join one of the road sidewalks and cross the bridge to Vacation Isle. Whether on vacation or not, this is a lovely little spot for on-foot exercise.

Continue along Ingraham Street across the second bridge. Get to the left side of the road. At the intersection with Dana Landing Road and Perez Cove Way, take the street to the left then pick up the paved bike trail past Sea World.

From this point on, follow our directions for the second half of the Sea World and Old Town route. Enjoy Old Town as a destination and use the Trolley to get back downtown.

# Other Ideas

There is a route around the **east part of Mission Bay Park**, including Fiesta Bay and Fiesta Island. However, the beauty and overall pleasantness of this area are so overshadowed by that of Mission Bay Park west that we could not recommend it. In particular, the northern edge of the bay on the east side takes you into very ordinary residential areas with no beauty at all. People do run around Fiesta Island but it is not particularly attractive. The eastern edge of the bay is quite pleasant but devoid of major attractions. Even the "Visitor's Center," billed as such on maps, highway signs, and the sign over the door, was a bit of a disappointment. After lining up there, seeking maps and visitor information, we were told, "We're not really a Visitor's Center!" So don't bother going in there. However, if you are a runner, you will find notices of all forthcoming running events at the Runners' Bathroom on the shore just south of the Visitor's Center.

Nola and I spent a memorable day in **Tecolote Canyon Natural Park**. It is a very interesting place—a natural wildlife area very close to the city, and reachable on foot from the Trolley Blue Line. However, we concluded it just does not meet our route selection criteria. The underfoot conditions were not generally very good, and signs warn of very real dangers such as rattlesnakes, poison oak, and mountain lions. It is not easy to find a route that is clearly defined and has a good destination. However, if you like wandering in the wilds over wildflower-abundant hilltops for a day, this might be for you.

**Torrey Pines**, on the ocean shore about 15 miles north of downtown, is a beautiful and popular park with a variety of on-foot trails. However, it is not really convenient to the city or public transit. If you have a car and day to spare, drive there, hike the trails, and drive back.

* * * *

San Diego has the best weather in the country for outdoor activities of any kind including running, jogging, and walking. It also has some gorgeous scenic views and some interesting historic sites, based on its origins as the first European settlement in California. As described in this chapter, there are some excellent pedestrian trails not far from the center of the city.

Put all this together and you have a formula for some very motivating and enjoyable time out on foot, here in the bottom-left corner of the 48 states. Have fun!

# 16

# Conclusion

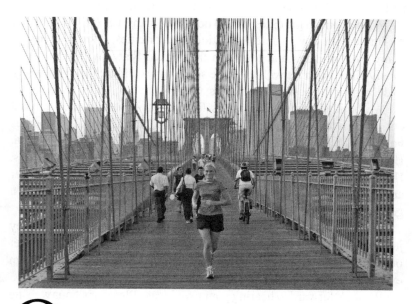

O ur tour is over.[1] We certainly enjoyed our time out on-foot in all 14 cities, while getting to know and appreciate those cities. We hope you will enjoy at least some of these places, as we did. Also, we hope we have helped encourage you to spend more time out on foot if you live in one of these cities or visit any of them.

We are often asked which city we think is the best for on-foot exercise. We have thought long and hard about this and concluded that there is no best city overall. Rather, different cities are best in different respects. Here is our assessment of some of the "bests":

---

1        Photo:  Louisa Ford on the Brooklyn Bridge.

Best trail system:  Minneapolis
Most interesting routes:  Washington
Most scenic routes:  San Francisco
Best weather:  San Diego
Best public transit:  Washington
Friendliest city:  Seattle and Indianapolis (a tie)

In making these calls, we are not implying that the other cities are particularly deficient.  For a city to make our cut for this book at all, it had to have admirable on-foot exercise qualities overall.

What about all the cities we did not cover in this book?  Well, firstly, we limited our coverage to the nation's major cities.  I know there are many smaller cities and towns in the United States with routes that satisfy all our criteria well.  Maybe some day we'll get the opportunity to document the best of those cities and towns.

We omitted some major cities for a conscious reason.  We ruled out cities with an average maximum temperature above 80 degrees Fahrenheit for six or more months of the year.  This cut Miami, Tampa, Houston, Phoenix, San Antonio, and some other southern places.  However, please enjoy your on-foot exercise in these cities in winter and in early mornings.  We omitted a couple of cities because of a generally bad reputation safety-wise.

For other major cities, we offer no excuse for their omission.  They just did not happen to make it up our priority list high enough to garner our attention.  I guess we just don't have enough hours to travel and run everywhere.  (Sigh...)

We look forward to hearing your own ideas.  Please visit our website www.funonfoot.com to provide your feedback.

And don't forget to have fun!

# About the Author(s)

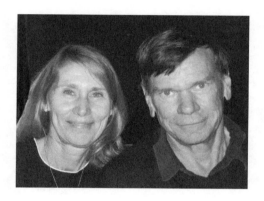

Warwick Ford and Nola Ford are Australian-raised Canadian-American travel addicts. As a Massachusetts-based executive of a California company, Warwick spent many years logging flight miles and visiting U.S. cities. One of the biggest challenges of that period was finding the motivation and the time to get out on-foot enough to maintain fitness. That led to this project. Now, Warwick and Nola spend time researching and documenting premium, enjoyable on-foot routes in cities throughout the United States and internationally. Warwick's previous titles were in the technology realm; they include *Computer Communications Security* and *Secure Electronic Commerce*, published by Prentice Hall PTR.